Praise .

Take Charge of Your Child's Sleep:
The All-in-One Resource for Solving Sleep Problems
in Kids and Teens

"This easy-to-follow 'how-to' book is a gold mine of information on sleep as it relates to youngsters. If your child or teen has a sleep problem, look to Drs. Owens and Mindell for proven solutions!"
—Dr. James Maas, Weiss Presidential Fellow/Professor, Cornell University and author of *Power Sleep*

"With this book, Drs. Owens and Mindell have filled a crucial need. A beacon of hope for a largely overlooked population, it provides solid advice to kids and teens who can't sleep and the parents who anguish over them."
—Tamar Chansky, PhD, author of *Freeing Your Child from Anxiety* and *Freeing Your Child from Obsessive-Compulsive Disorder*

Judith A. Owens, MD, a developmental-behavioral pediatrician, is the director of the Pediatric Sleep Disorders Clinic and the Learning, Attention, and Behavior Clinic at Hasbro Children's Hospital in Providence, Rhode Island.

Jodi A. Mindell, PhD, author of *Sleeping Through the Night: How Infants, Toddlers, and Their Parents Can Get a Good Night's Sleep,* is the associate director of the Sleep Center at The Children's Hospital of Philadelphia and professor of psychology at Saint Joseph's University.

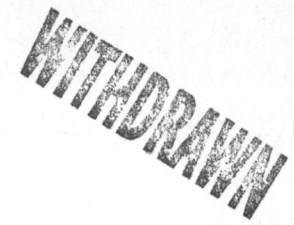

TAKE CHARGE OF YOUR CHILD'S SLEEP:

The All-in-One Resource for Solving Sleep Problems in Kids and Teens

Judy A. Owens, MD, and
Jodi A. Mindell, PhD

MARLOWE & COMPANY
NEW YORK

Published by
Marlowe & Company
An Imprint of Avalon Publishing Group Incorporated
245 West 17th Street • 11th floor
New York, NY 10011

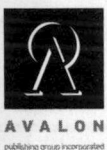

AVALON
publishing group incorporated

ISBN-13: 978-1-56924-362-6

Library of Congress Cataloging-in-Publication Data
Owens, Judith A.
  Take charge of your child's sleep: the all-in-one resource for solving sleep problems in kids and teens / Judith Owens and Jodi Mindell.
    p.cm.
  Includes bibliographical references and index.
  ISBN 1-56924-362-X (trade pbk.)
  1. Sleep disorders in children—Popular works. I. Mindell, Jodi A. II. Title.
    RJ506.S55O945 2005
    618.92'8498—dc22

9 8 7 6 5 4 3 2

Interior design by Maria E. Torres

Printed in the United States of America

The information in this book is intended to help readers make informed decisions about their health and the health of their loved ones. It is not intended to be a substitute for treatment by or the advice and care of a professional health care provider. While the authors and publisher have endeavored to ensure that the information presented is accurate and up to date, they are not responsible for adverse effects or consequences sustained by any person using this book.

To Thad, Evan, and Grace

To Scott and Caelie

Contents

PART ONE: THE BASICS OF SLEEP

1

The Top Ten Reasons
Why a Good Night's Sleep Is Important

Sleep is *the* main occupation of children and adolescents, starting right from birth. By age two, the average baby has spent an impressive 9,500 hours (or a total of thirteen months) in dreamland, in contrast to 8,000 hours in all other activities combined. Between the ages of two and five, a child spends approximately equal amounts of time awake and asleep. And throughout childhood and adolescence, sleep accounts for about 40 percent of a child's day.

However, despite the vital role that Mother Nature has obviously assigned to sleep, the importance of healthy sleep and the consequences of not getting enough sleep are often overlooked by parents, teachers, coaches, doctors, and everyone else who cares for and about children and adolescents. So why the disconnect? Clearly, there are many reasons for this state of affairs. First, technological advances like ATM machines and the Internet have made a "24/7" society possible. Activities that used to occur only during the day, like shopping and banking, are now possible at all times of the day and night. Basically, you can do just about anything in the middle of the night that you can do during the day. The consequences of this "brave new world" range from parents whose work schedules span the clock to the twenty-four-hour "cartoon channel." And few children, when faced with the lure of *Scooby Doo* reruns at 11:00 PM would choose *to go to sleep!* Furthermore, the modern parent's mantra of "quality time," combined with our workaholic "sleep is for slackers" mentality, often results in sleep being squeezed out of the list of daily priorities.

However, just as no parent would allow their child to exist solely on a diet of french fries and soda, every parent also has the responsibility to make healthy sleep happen for their child or teen. Like good nutrition, seatbelts, and SPF 30 suntan lotion, a good night's sleep is a necessary part of a healthy lifestyle, and it is in the best interest of your child. What's more, it also directly benefits you as a parent. After all, it's the rare mom or dad who would actually choose to deal with the "sleepy, dopey, and grumpy" syndrome when they could have a cheerful and well-rested child. Furthermore, by getting those critical eight hours of zzz's yourself, you might even find that you don't need that double-espresso latte every morning to get your own batteries recharged!

Still not convinced that the nagging needed to get your eight-year-old to turn off the TV and go to bed, or the amount of persuasion it would take to get your teen to turn in at a reasonable hour, is worth the hassle? Well, here (with apologies to David Letterman) are the "Top Ten Reasons Why a Good Night's Sleep Is Important":

Reason #1: Poor sleep is one of the most common problems of children and adolescents.

There are few pediatric health issues that are more common than childhood sleep disorders. Most studies report that about 25 percent of all children experience some type of sleep problem at some point during childhood and adolescence. These range from short-term problems such as falling asleep and waking at night (see chapters 8 and 9) to more serious sleep disorders such as obstructive sleep apnea and narcolepsy (see chapters 13 and 16). Snoring occurs in about 10 percent of preschool-aged children; while obstructive sleep apnea, a serious breathing problem, affects at least three in every one hundred children. A recent poll by the National Sleep Foundation found that 69 percent of parents of children ages ten and under reported that their child had at least one sleep problem a few nights a week. And almost three out of four parents wanted to change something about their child's sleep! As for older kids, not only do the vast majority of adolescents not get enough sleep, but close to half of all teens also complain of sleep problems, such as insomnia.

Finally, not getting enough sleep and sleep problems are becoming even more common. For example, the number of adolescents who report being chronically sleepy during the day has risen significantly over the past few decades. And the amount of sleep that children of all ages are now getting has steadily decreased since the 1970s.

Reason #2: Childhood sleep problems can be chronic.

Although many sleep problems in children are short-lived, the common wisdom that children "grow out of" sleep problems is usually not true. Some sleep problems continue into or resurface in adulthood. Other chronic sleep disorders, such as restless legs syndrome and narcolepsy (see chapters 14 and 16), may first start in childhood or adolescence. In addition, there are circumstances that may make it more likely for a child to develop a chronic sleep problem. For example, a child with a chronic illness or with developmental delays is more likely to continue to have sleep issues. Parent-related and family-related problems, such as maternal depression and a high level of family stress, also make it more likely that small, short-term sleep problems will hang around long enough to become big ones.

Reason #3: Sleep problems in children are highly treatable.

Now for the good news—sleep problems can be treated. Many highly effective treatments for sleep disorders in children and adolescents are available. In addition, researchers are continuing to develop new and better ones.

Not only does treatment of a sleep problem make nighttime better, but you will also notice a huge difference in your child during the day. For example, removing the tonsils and adenoids of a child who has obstructive sleep apnea can lead to major improvements in that child's mood, behavior, and school performance.

Reason #4: Sleep problems are preventable.

Sleep problems are not only treatable, but they are also preventable. Parents can learn strategies to prevent sleep problems from developing in the first place, as well as from becoming chronic if they already exist. For example, setting a regular bedtime and bedtime routine for your preschooler, developing good sleep habits for your middle-schooler, and knowing the amount of sleep your teenager *needs* (but does not often *get!*)

can go a long way toward avoiding bedtime struggles, miserable mornings, and dozing off in the classroom.

Reason #5: Sleep problems in children have a major impact on the whole family.

Sleep problems are often a big source of stress and distress for families. Every sleep problem in a child is automatically a problem for a parent (and often for his or her siblings, grandparents, and anyone else living in the house). Also, children's sleep problems often have a direct effect on parents' sleep. This results in caregivers who are exhausted, irritable, and less likely to be effective parents during the day. The flip side of this is that successful treatment can improve the sleep of your entire family, not just your child.

Reason #6: Sleep problems are one of the most frequent concerns that parents raise with their child's health care provider.

One study of pediatricians found that nearly 25 percent of their patients between the ages of six months and four years had sleep problems that were brought up by parents. Sleep concerns were ranked as the fifth leading parental concern, following illness, feeding, behavior problems, and physical abnormalities.

However, parents don't always recognize when their child has a sleep problem. Or if they do, they may not think to raise the issue to their pediatrician. This is especially true when their child is past the toddler years. At the same time, most pediatricians don't even question parents of older children and teens about sleep issues. They figure that if there is a problem, the parent will bring it up. The end result of this "conspiracy of silence" is that many important sleep issues are never addressed.

Reason #7: Sleep is necessary for children's optimal functioning.

A wealth of important research, much of it conducted in the past decade, clearly indicates that children and adolescents have significant daytime sleepiness as a result of not getting enough sleep or having poor sleep. This link between poor sleep and being sleepy the next day sounds like it should be pretty obvious. However, the research also shows that this daytime sleepiness leads to major behavior problems and poor school performance. For example, one area of research has looked at how children do after sleeping less than normal amounts for several nights in a row. In one study, researchers had middle-school-aged children sleep only six and a half hours every night for a week. They found that this led to significant learning problems, such as poor attention span, difficulty with problem solving, and decreased speed and efficiency in completing tasks. So get your child to bed on time, especially on school nights!

Other studies have looked at children who were described by their parents as being "poor sleepers" or who had a known sleep disorder, such as obstructive sleep apnea. These children had more severe behavioral issues and mood problems compared to children without sleep problems. It is also well known that children with obstructive sleep apnea often have significant school performance problems.

Still other studies have examined the reverse situation. What does the sleep of children who already have a mood, behavioral, and/or academic problem, such as attention-deficit/hyperactivity disorder (ADHD) look like? Not surprisingly, these children experience more sleep problems than other children. Not getting enough sleep and sleep problems are also related to adolescents and college students doing poorly in school. Thus, it is clear that poor sleep goes hand in hand with poor learning, behavior, and school performance.

The term "optimal functioning" deserves further comment. Many adults are convinced that they (and their children) can get by on less sleep than the eight-plus hours most of us "grown-ups" (Donald Trump notwithstanding) need. There are several problems with this reasoning. First, most human beings are notoriously poor at judging how impaired they (and others) are from lack of sleep. And in fact they tend to underestimate the degree to which their performance is compromised. Furthermore, the sleepier you are, the less likely you are to recognize problems with how you are functioning. Second, sleep deprivation often initially affects more subtle "higher level" aspects of thinking and behavior, such as creative thought and attention span. These are the very things that can ultimately make the difference between your child's academic success and failure. Finally, when you think of it, no parent is likely to voluntarily withhold other things that would help their child improve their chances for success. So it makes just as much good sense to give your child the advantage of a good night's sleep as it does to provide a healthy breakfast, help with homework, or to choose the best possible school in order to help him succeed.

Reason #8: Sleep affects every aspect of a child's health and development.

We are just beginning to understand the negative effects in children of not getting enough sleep or getting a poor night's sleep. Overall, sleep affects every aspect of a child's physical, emotional, cognitive, and social development. Every parent knows that mood problems in children who are not sleeping well or not sleeping enough are virtually universal. A child is cranky, irritable, and whiny after a poor night's sleep, and his ability to regulate his mood may be affected. Children may also have problems with attention, hyperactivity, and poor impulse control. These problems not only affect school performance, but can also have an effect on a child's ability to socialize—that is, how well he interacts with his friends, teachers, and family members.

Equally important is the fact that sleep affects a child's health. Not getting enough sleep leads to more accidents, ranging from minor injuries to teens falling asleep at the wheel and having drowsy-driving accidents. There are also potential negative effects on a child's cardiovascular, immune, and metabolic systems. For example, young children with obstructive sleep apnea are more likely to have growth problems. In addition, chronic sleep deprivation is thought to possibly play a role in the development of obesity, now at epidemic levels in children in the United States. New evidence linking poor immune function to not getting enough sleep may eventually prove Mom's sage warning that "if you don't get enough sleep, you'll get sick!" was right on the money.

Reason #9: Sleep problems can make virtually any medical, emotional, or developmental problem worse.

Because poor sleep affects both our health and ability to function the next day, any medical or mental health problem is likely to be made worse by a sleep problem. Furthermore, sleep problems themselves tend to be more common in children and adolescents with chronic medical and psychiatric conditions. Thus, the behavior of a child with ADHD will be worse.

Depression in an adolescent will be more severe. Chronic pain conditions like juvenile rheumatoid arthritis are exacerbated. And parent-child conflicts are more problematic when sleep is poor. Conversely, improving sleep will have major benefits in these children as well.

Reason #10: Sleep is a public health problem.

While it may seem odd to include sleep problems and inadequate sleep with other public health issues like smoking and heart disease, the financial burden alone of childhood sleep problems is considerable. For example, the economic cost of visits to a health care professional for infant crying and sleeping problems is the equivalent of $104 million a year! Another recent study found a 200 percent increase in health care use, including increased hospital days, drugs, and emergency room visits, in children with obstructive sleep apnea.

Despite this, surveys suggest that pediatric health care providers often do not adequately address sleep issues. In a recent survey of pediatricians, almost a quarter of the physicians did not routinely screen for sleep problems in school-aged children during well-child visits. In addition, only 25 percent asked about snoring in preschoolers, and less than 40 percent questioned adolescents about their sleep habits. This was despite the same physicians' acknowledging that sleep is important and has a major impact on health, behavior, and school performance. In contrast, in a survey of early adolescents, the students themselves identified their health care provider as one of the most important and reliable sources of information about healthy sleep (although most of them also said that their doctor never asks them about their sleep!).

For all those reasons and more . . .

Hopefully you had a hunch even before reading this chapter that sleep is important, or, if not, our top ten list has helped you "see the light." Sleep should clearly be a critical part of your child's days for the very good reasons listed above. But even if you have been slacking off a bit in the parent sleep-patrol department, don't despair—help is on the way! Most importantly, realize that major changes are not always necessary to give your child a good night's sleep. Relatively small changes, such as moving your child's bedtime thirty minutes earlier or stopping him from drinking a large caffeine-filled soft drink at 7:00 PM, can make a huge difference for your child—and for you!

So do yourself and your child a very big favor by making sleep a priority for her and for your entire family. Let us show you how to develop a sleep plan that not only meets your child's needs, but also suits his "sleep personality" (see chapter 2) and fits with the way your family works. You will be giving your child a gift of a lifetime . . . or at least of a nighttime!

2

Sleep 101: Straight Talk about Sleep and Sleep Problems in Kids

What is sleep, anyway? First, sleep is not just the opposite of being awake. Sleep is also not a passive state in which nothing happens. And it is most decidedly not just a waste of time.

Sleep is actually a very active and busy time for both the brain and the body. Many important biological processes occur during sleep. Almost every system in the body you can think of is active during sleep. For example, during rapid eye movement (REM) or "dream" sleep, the brain is just as active as it is when fully awake. There are also important biological processes that occur almost exclusively when we are asleep. For instance, the majority of human growth hormone, which is essential for normal growth in children, is released during sleep.

In addition, sleep can be thought of as both a biological process and a learned behavior. That sounds like a contradiction, doesn't it? How can sleep be a normal biological function of the body that goes on all the time without our even thinking about it (as with breathing, digesting food, and fighting infections) but at the same time be something we can learn to control? Especially since, when we're sleeping, we aren't even aware of what's going on around us?

Well, when you think about it, it's really not so different from what happens with most of the other normal functions of the body. Like sleep, those other functions are also affected by what goes on both in our heads and all around us. For example, breathing is a normal biological function, but we can consciously speed it up or slow it down. We can help our body fight an infection, such as a cold, by getting lots of sleep and drinking plenty of liquids. Ditto with sleep. Sleep can be affected by what we drink (think Starbucks), what's going on around us (an exciting sports event versus a boring lecture), and our physical environment (too hot, too noisy). It is clear that how and when we sleep, while "hard-wired" by biology, is also affected by many other factors.

Because children and teenagers are still growing and developing, their sleep patterns and sleep habits are still developing as well. This makes it even more important for parents to start as early as possible to help their children develop good sleep habits, and to continue to support (and model!) good sleep throughout childhood and adolescence. Each child has a unique "sleep personality" that starts with biology (the common biological processes that regulate sleep in all of us). But children's sleep personalities are also influenced and shaped by many other factors, such as the genes they inherit from their parents, what they learn from parents and other adults, their early experiences, their environment, and even what lullabies you sang to them when they were babies. Ask yourself these simple questions to help figure out your child's "sleep personality."

WHAT IS YOUR CHILD'S "SLEEP PERSONALITY"?

- How much sleep does your child need to feel "well-rested"?

- How sensitive is your child to not getting as much sleep as he needs?

- What is your child like when she hasn't gotten enough sleep?

- What time does your child prefer to go to bed at night and get up in the morning?

- How much "calm down" time does your child need before bed?

- What relaxes your child at bedtime?

- What makes your child feel "safe" at night?

- How difficult is it for your child to get back to sleep if she wakes up at night?

- What is your child like first thing in the morning?

Sleep Architecture: The Building Blocks

From a sleep scientist's perspective, there are basically three very separate states of being in which all of us spend our lives: (1) awake, (2) REM (rapid eye movement) sleep, and (3) non-REM sleep. Each of these states involves different parts of the brain and different brain chemicals, known as *neurotransmitters*. Each of these three states is unique, although there is some overlap. For example, our brains are very active when we are awake and during REM sleep. During REM sleep and non-REM sleep, our brains are clearly sleeping. Surprisingly, REM sleep and non-REM sleep are as different from one another as the difference between being awake and asleep.

The building blocks that make up the basic structure of these states are called *sleep stages*. This is also referred to as *sleep architecture*. Each sleep stage is unique in its pattern of brain waves (electroencephalogram or EEG) and body movements, particularly eye movements. The sleep stages also differ in the level of awareness of the sleeper and how easy, or difficult, it is to wake him.

Non-REM sleep. Non-REM sleep is divided into four separate stages.

- **Stage 1.** Stage 1 is a kind of brief "transition" sleep between wake and stage 2. It usually takes up only about 2–5 percent of the night. People are easily awakened from stage 1 sleep, and may not even realize they have been asleep. Sleep starts or "nap jerks" are common, and some people experience short periods of feeling like they are paralyzed as they drift off to sleep.
- **Stage 2.** Stage 2 sleep is usually considered the beginning of "true" sleep and on an average night makes up the greatest portion of the night (50 percent). You can be easily awakened from stage 2, but you are clearly asleep.
- **Stages 3 and 4.** Stages 3 and 4 together are known as *deep sleep, slow wave sleep,* or *delta sleep.* Breathing and heart rate are very slow and regular during these stages. It is very difficult to awaken someone from deep sleep. When your child is in deep sleep, you can pick him up, change his clothes, and put him to bed without him ever waking up. When people sleep through earthquakes or don't

hear the phone ringing, they are usually in deep sleep. This stage of sleep is considered the most restful or "restorative" stage. If someone is not sleeping enough, then a greater percentage of his sleep will be deep sleep in order to compensate for the smaller amount of sleep he is getting. *Recovery sleep,* or the sleep that occurs after being sleep deprived, also has a greater than normal percent of deep sleep. This is also the stage of sleep in which sleepwalking and sleep terrors occur. The amount of deep sleep is highest in early childhood (50 percent of sleep), drops during adolescence, and then continues to decrease to a very small percentage (3–5 percent) in elderly people. This seems to indicate that there is something fundamental to growth and development about this particular type of sleep.

REM sleep. REM sleep was discovered almost exactly fifty years ago. A sleep researcher named Nathaniel Kleitman noticed that frequent fast (rapid) eye movements were very prominent during active sleep in young babies. REM sleep is also commonly known as "dream sleep," because it is the stage of sleep in which dreaming largely (though not exclusively) takes place.

REM sleep is a very active type of sleep. Your brain waves during REM sleep look very much as they do when you are awake. Another unique feature of REM sleep is that virtually all of the muscles in the body (except for those that control breathing) are paralyzed during this stage of sleep. This essentially prevents us from "acting out" our dreams.

In adults, REM sleep occupies roughly 20–25 percent of a typical night's sleep. In contrast, newborns spend about half of their time asleep in REM-like or what is referred to as *active sleep.* This again suggests that there is something about REM sleep that is essential during the developmental process in early childhood.

Sleep Cycles: What Goes Around Comes Around

Sleep also has a very set structure in terms of the timing (cycles) of the sleep stages throughout the night. Non-REM and REM sleep alternate about every

90–110 minutes in adults. The first ninety minutes or so is all non-REM sleep. After ninety minutes, a period of REM sleep will occur, followed by a return to non-REM sleep. After that, about every ninety minutes a REM period will occur. The first REM periods of the night are quite short, lasting just a few minutes, and get longer as the night goes on. In children, a sleep cycle is much shorter. It starts at about every fifty minutes or so in infants and gradually increases through childhood to adult lengths.

What is most important about these sleep cycles is that most of them will end in a short period of awakening from sleep, or a partial awakening called an *arousal,* before the sleeper goes on to the next sleep cycle. So in very young children, these short arousals occur as a matter of course at about sixty- to ninety-minute intervals, up to ten times a night. Fortunately, these are normally followed by an equally rapid return to dreamland, until the next sleep cycle ends. But in those children who have never learned to fall asleep by themselves, these brief arousals can rapidly escalate into full-blown, middle-of-the-night distress calls for parental assistance. So it's not the *waking* that's the problem, it's the not-being-able-to-fall-back-asleep-on-my-own that is the real culprit.

The other important thing to understand about sleep cycles, as mentioned above, is that the amount of slow wave sleep decreases and REM increases over the course of the night. The result is that most slow wave sleep occurs in the first third of the night and most REM sleep in the last third. Thus, sleep behaviors that are associated with deep sleep (like sleepwalking) are more likely to occur in the early part of the night, while things that happened during REM sleep (like nightmares) happen more often toward the early morning hours.

Who's in Charge Here?: What Controls Sleep

We are just beginning to have a true understanding of the very complicated biological processes that determine when we are awake and when we are asleep. The systems that control sleep have their origins in the brain and involve neurotransmitters (chemical messengers). But the regulation of sleep is also influenced by many other factors, including all of the many things that compete with sleep for our time.

Sleep Regulation: Clocks and Thermostats

The two major systems involved in the control of sleep are called the *sleep drive* and the *sleep* or *circadian clock*. Both of these systems act at the same time. Sometimes they work together (in the same direction), and sometimes they act in opposition to each other. How sleepy or how awake you are at any given time is the result of the combined forces of the sleep drive and sleep clock.

Sleep drive. The sleep drive acts sort of like a thermostat for sleep. As you might imagine, the sleep drive is very dependent upon how long you have been awake and how much sleep (and what quality) you got the night before. It starts out at a very low level when you wake up in the morning and then builds steadily over the course of the day (unless you take a nap), with the drive or pressure to sleep becoming stronger the longer you are up. Once you've gotten your appropriate quota of a good night's sleep, the sleep drive returns to a very low level.

Sleep clock. The sleep clock (circadian clock), on the other hand, is a regular internal rhythm of sleep and wake that is controlled by a specific area of the brain (called the *suprachiasmatic nucleus,* for those of you who like to know these things). There are two periods of maximum sleepiness and two periods of maximum wakefulness during the twenty-four-hour day. The periods of peak sleepiness occur in the late afternoon (3:00–5:00 PM; siesta time!) and in the middle of the night (3:00–5:00 AM, when most of us are already asleep). The two periods of peak alertness happen in the early to mid-morning and in mid to late evening (commonly known as the "second wind").

The sleep clock is also affected by cues in the environment that help keep it on a twenty-four-hour time course. These cues include the timing of daily activities and, most important, exposure to light. Light influences the circadian clock by switching off the body's production of the hormone *melatonin*. Melatonin, which is normally turned on in the evening and turned off in the morning, is one of the body's most powerful sleep messengers. So exposure to light in the evening slows the body's production of melatonin and makes it more difficult to fall asleep. The same effect of light exposure on melatonin in the morning has the helpful effect of waking you up.

The Bottom Line: Why We Sleep

The funny thing is, despite the explosion of information in the past fifty years about what sleep is and how we do it, exactly *why* we sleep remains pretty much a mystery. What we do know is what happens when people (or any living creature, for that matter) don't sleep. For example, the brain slows down, the immune system starts to malfunction, and the body's metabolism starts to go haywire. And we know that sleep deprivation, if it goes on long enough, can be fatal. So it's pretty safe to conclude that sleep is necessary for us to thrive and survive.

Beyond that, we have only theories about the true function of sleep. Some scientists view sleep as an opportunity to sort through, process, and make sense of all the information we take in during the day, as well as to decide what stays and what goes (memory). Other theories state that sleep is important in restoring the body and repairing the physical wear and tear of daily life. The reality is that there are probably multiple reasons why sleep is just as important to us as breathing and eating. When you think about it, why else would it make sense that human beings evolved to spend a third of their lives doing something that makes them much more vulnerable to being eaten by the nearest wild animal?

When Good Sleep Goes Bad: What Causes Sleep Problems

Sleep problems are basically what happens when one or more of these complicated brain systems that control sleep has a malfunction or gets derailed. This can happen in several different ways:

- **The amount of sleep you get is not enough to meet your sleep needs.** Insufficient sleep, especially in older children and adolescents, can be the result of a conscious lifestyle decision to sacrifice sleep in favor of the competition, such as extracurricular/social activities and after-school jobs. Insufficient sleep can also result from difficulty falling asleep, staying asleep, or from waking up too early in the morning.
- **The quality of sleep is poor.** Children can get the right amount of sleep, but the quality of their sleep is poor. For example, their sleep may be interrupted by wakings during the night or may not be

restful. Sleep disorders that briefly disturb sleep repeatedly throughout the night, such as obstructive sleep apnea, often result in poor sleep quality.

- **There is a problem falling asleep or staying asleep.** There are many reasons why a child has a problem falling asleep or staying asleep. It could be a behavioral issue, such as resisting going to bed or waking up at night and needing a parent nearby in order to fall back to sleep (see chapters 8 and 9). It could also be the result of sleep problems like insomnia or restless legs syndrome (see chapters 11 and 14).
- **The timing of sleep is off or conflicts with the rest of what you need to do.** In this situation, the amount and quality of the sleep is not a problem, but *when it happens* is. This most commonly occurs in teenagers whose internal clocks are set to fall asleep later and wake up later but whose external alarm clocks are telling them it's time to get up (see chapter 15).
- **There is some imbalance in the body between sleep and wakefulness.** Although not common, this kind of imbalance occurs in sleep disorders like narcolepsy, and usually results in severe daytime sleepiness (chapter 16).
- **There are things going on during sleep that shouldn't be.** The category of sleep problems known as *parasomnias* (nightmares, sleep terrors, and sleepwalking) involve the interruption of normal sleep by odd behaviors or by behaviors that don't usually happen during sleep. Because they mostly occur while someone is asleep, parasomnias are often less disturbing to the sleeper than they are to the person observing them. (See chapters 10 and 12 for more information on these sleep problems.)

Sometimes there is more than one culprit. For example, children with obstructive sleep apnea have frequent interruptions (arousals) during sleep caused by breathing pauses. These arousals can trigger a parasomnia, such as sleepwalking. Teenagers with a sleep-wake pattern that is delayed (later than normal) often also have insufficient sleep, because they still have to get up early in the morning.

So Doctor, How Do I Know if My Child Has a Sleep Problem?

Some sleep problems are immediately obvious to parents, such as sleep-walking and bedtime resistance. Others may not be so obvious, such as periodic limb movement disorder. But since sleep problems can have very significant consequences for children's health and functioning, it is very important for parents to know and recognize the symptoms of a possible sleep problem in their child or teenager. The best way to deal with most sleep problems is to find them early and treat them as soon as possible. That way, little sleep problems are much less likely to become big (or even lifelong)

BEARS

We have developed a simple set of sleep questions for parents called the BEARS. Each letter stands for a different potential sleep problem area. Ask yourself the following questions to help identify sleep issues that might be a concern in your child.

B = Bedtime

> Does your child have difficulty going to bed? Falling asleep?

E = Excessive daytime sleepiness

> Is your child always difficult to wake up in the morning?

> Does your child seem sleepy or groggy during the day?

> Does he or she often seem overtired (this can mean moody, "hyper, " or "out of it" as well as sleepy)?

A = Awakenings during the night

> Does your child wake up at night? Have trouble falling back to sleep?

> Does anything else seem to interrupt his sleep?

R = Regularity and amount of sleep

S = Snoring

> Does your child snore? Loudly? Every night? Does he ever stop breathing or choke or gasp during sleep?

A yes answer to one of more of these questions could mean that your child has a sleep problem that should be looked into further. More details about each of these potential sleep problem areas can be found in Part Three: Sleep Problems and Solutions.

3

Sleep Across the Ages: What's Normal and What's Not

E very parent at one time or another has asked "Is this normal?" about their child's behavior. Comparing your child's behavior to that of other children the same age is natural and oftentimes reassuring (even if it doesn't necessarily make the behavior any easier to live with!). The same principle certainly applies to sleep. It's very helpful as a parent to know what's "normal." Finding out what's normal can help you decide if you should be worried about whether your son or daughter is getting enough sleep, should be waking up at night, or is experiencing other sleep issues, like falling asleep in school

The trouble is, "normal" doesn't necessarily mean "good." We know, for example, that the typical teenager in the United States gets a little over seven hours of sleep a night. But the average teenager needs more like nine hours of sleep. So in this case, the norm is far from ideal, and, in fact, it's not even close to okay. To make things more complicated, we're not always sure what either "normal" or "the ideal" is when it comes to many aspects of children's sleep. Sometimes we don't know because the research hasn't gotten that far. Other times it's because the definition depends on who's asking. For example, in most Asian cultures it's perfectly acceptable and "normal" to still have your five- or six- or seven-year-old sleeping in the same bed with you. In the United States, however, this practice would probably raise at least some eyebrows, and might even be frowned upon by some child psychologists.

All that having been said, there are some reasonable expectations that parents should have about what constitutes normal sleep at different developmental stages in childhood. The current best estimates of normal sleep amounts and descriptions of sleep patterns in various age groups are outlined below. Ranges for sleep amounts at each age are also listed, based on studies of sleep patterns in large groups of children. The smaller number is the amount of sleep reported for those 2 percent of children at that age who get the least amount of sleep and the higher number is the sleep amount reported for those 2 percent of children who get the most amount of sleep. Also included are age-specific developmental changes that can have an important influence on sleep, common sleep issues, and some of the most frequent sleep problems that occur at different ages.

Preschoolers (3 to 5 years)

Timothy is four years old. He goes to bed every night at 8:00, although he usually spends another half-hour repeatedly calling for his parents after lights-out. He still takes a two-hour nap on most days, although many of his friends have stopped napping. Timothy sleeps with a stuffed monkey, which he is sure keeps the monsters away at night.

The Numbers

- **Average hours of sleep:** 11 to 12 hours over 24 hours
  Range: $9\frac{1}{2}$ to $14\frac{1}{2}$ hours
  Naps: Children stop taking naps at different ages. Most children stop napping between the ages of three and four, but many children continue to nap up to the age of six.

PERCENTAGE OF CHILDREN STILL TAKING NAPS	
AGE	PERCENT STILL NAPPING
3 years	92%
4 years	57%
5 years	27%

10/29/2021

JACKSON LAUREN E

Item Number: 31901046184968

Items may be renewed online at
http://ccclib.org or by calling 1-800-984-4636,
menu option 1. Book drops will be open for
returns. Ygnacio Valley Library remains
temporarily closed.

Hold Shelf Slip

Developmental Issues and Sleep

As with everything else, different aspects of development will affect your child's sleep. Below are some common developmental aspects of the preschool years and how they affect sleep.

- **Testing of limits.** As preschoolers develop more thinking skills, and become more aware of rules and limits and of what's expected of them, they may also do more testing of those limits. This can lead to pushing the envelope when it comes to bedtime rules. You may find that your child, now that he is a preschooler, struggles more and resists going to sleep when it's time for lights-out.
- **Language.** As their language becomes more sophisticated, children also become better able to tell you what they want. They also develop more creative ways of expressing themselves. One effect of these growing language skills is the seemingly endless parade of "curtain calls" at bedtime (another story, drink, kiss, hug) that parents are often subjected to at this age.
- **Imagination.** Preschoolers are very imaginative creatures. However, they are not always able to separate their fantasies from the facts. For the same reason that Santa Claus and the tooth fairy are so popular at this age, the boogeyman and monsters under the bed (in the closet, outside the window) are equally real. Nighttime fears are fairly universal at this age. The key is learning how to handle them so that little monsters don't become big ones (see chapter 10).
- **Understanding consequences.** Children at this age are starting to develop the ability to understand the consequences of their behavior. They are now able to wait a short time for rewards (delayed gratification). They also really want to please grown-ups in general, and parents in particular. Reward systems (this is the Golden Age of Sticker Charts) and lots of praise can often be a parent's best ally in managing bedtime battles (see chapter 8).
- **Reading at bedtime.** As children become more interested in reading and books, the value of reading aloud at bedtime as part of

the bedtime routine becomes increasingly important in helping them to develop literacy skills. That nightly fifteen minutes of Dr. Seuss can help foster a lifetime love of reading!

Common Sleep Issues

There are a number of sleep issues that are common to the preschool years.

- **Naps.** Parents of preschoolers are often concerned about what's normal in terms of naps. As stated above, a large percentage of children stop napping between the ages of three and four. However, many children continue to nap up to age five and even beyond. The continued need for naps and the age at which your child is ready to give them up is part of your child's unique "sleep personality" (see chapter 2), and there are no hard and fast rules about this. The key is making sure that your child is well rested. Eliminating naps, if your child still needs one, will not help your child sleep better at night. On the other hand, napping too close to bedtime may interfere with falling asleep. There may often be a transition period of several months when your child still really needs her nap, but napping makes it difficult for her to fall asleep at bedtime. In this case, you should stick with her normal bedtime, but add thirty to forty-five minutes of quiet playtime in her bed before lights-out. If she calls you or comes out of her room, the light gets turned off. It usually takes only one time before your child realizes that it's worth quietly playing and not asking for you.
- **Sleep schedules.** Preschoolers need a set, consistent bedtime and wake time. A regular and consistent daytime routine (such as set mealtimes and playtimes) also helps to reinforce the sleep/wake schedule. There are no absolute rules about the "ideal" bedtime for children at this age, but you should base the schedule you set for your child on the amount of sleep he or she needs. For example, if your child attends afternoon kindergarten, he may do fine with a relatively later bed (and wake) time. Just keep in mind that you are going to have to readjust your child's sleep schedule eventually. When it's time to make the shift, be sure to start several

weeks in advance of the anticipated change so that the shift is not too abrupt. This same principle applies to shifting bedtime forward or backward when daylight savings time changes. Anticipating just this one-hour shift by a few days to a week or so and moving bedtime by ten to fifteen minutes a night in the appropriate direction makes for less of a fight in the evening and fewer cranky mornings!

- **Bedtime routines.** A bedtime routine is an important daily ritual that helps both children and adults. Bedtime routines help your child transition from a busy day to nighttime calm, from being in the middle of things to being alone in bed, and from wide-awake to fast asleep. At the end of the day, both the body and mind need to wind down, relax, and prepare physically and mentally for sleep. A bedtime routine is the best way to make sure there is enough time to make that transition. The ideal bedtime routine consists of a series of activities that are pleasant, relaxing, and the same every night (such as bath, pajamas, brush teeth, and story). The sameness of the routine will help to cue your child's body and mind that it is time for sleep.

BEDTIME ROUTINE TIPS

- Make the routine exactly the same every night.

- Incorporate three to four activities into your child's routine.

- Develop a routine that is enjoyable for you and your child.

- Don't let the routine keep heading in different directions—upstairs for a bath, to the kitchen for a snack, to the living room for a video, to the parent's room for a story, and finally to your child's room for hugs and kisses.

- Make the last part of your child's bedtime a special routine.

- Incorporate bedtime stories into your child's routine. They are a special way to connect and help develop a love of reading.

- **Transitional objects.** A lovey (more formally known as a *transitional object*) at bedtime and naptime, such as a special blanket, a doll, or a stuffed animal, is another important way in that you can help your preschooler make the leap from wake to sleep. Each child has his own version of Linus's famous blanket that makes him feel safe and secure. Sometimes parents worry about children becoming too dependent on a particular doll or stuffed toy, but transitional objects actually help children become *more* independent about getting themselves to sleep. Thumb sucking is another kind of transitional object that is highly convenient, always available, and doesn't have to go through the trauma of machine-washing. Before the age of four or so, especially if limited to bedtime, thumb sucking is unlikely to result in significant dental problems. (Please note: a television set is *not* a transitional object and has no place being in any child's bedroom or being a part of a preschooler's regular bedtime routine. More about this in chapter 5.)
- **The second wind.** The second wind or "forbidden zone" is the normal late-day surge in energy that most of us have in the early evening hours, but it may be exaggerated in some children. If you attempt to put your child to bed at a time when his sleep clock is saying "let's go!" loud and clear, you are likely to meet with a great deal of resistance and may have quite a struggle on your hands. Move your child's bedtime earlier or (horrors!) later. This avoids having it occur smack in the middle of the second wind and solves the problem of the child who is always wide-awake at bedtime.

Common Sleep Problems

- **Nighttime fears and nightmares.** As mentioned above, as your child's imagination develops, nighttime fears and nightmares are sure to follow. These two sleep issues are almost universal during the preschool years (see chapter 10).
- **Bedtime struggles.** Preschoolers are notorious for stalling at bedtime and resisting going to bed. By developing a consistent bedtime routine and setting limits at bedtime, you can both prevent and help solve bedtime issues (see chapter 8).

- **Night wakings.** Mostly we think of night wakings as being a problem only for infants and toddlers, but night wakings can easily continue into the preschool years (see chapter 9).
- **Obstructive sleep apnea.** Preschool is the time when children are at the highest risk for sleep apnea, given that is the time that the tonsils and adenoids are at their largest (the most common reason for sleep apnea in children). If your child snores, has breathing pauses, or seems to have any trouble breathing during the night, be sure to read chapter 13.
- **Sleepwalking and sleep terrors.** Sleepwalking and sleep terrors are also most commonly seen during the preschool years. It's not totally clear why this is, but it's likely because there is a high percentage of slow wave sleep (the sleep stage is when these events occur). (For more information on these two common sleep issues, see chapter 12.)

School-aged Children (6 to 12 years)

Sonya is nine years old and had always been a great sleeper. For the past six months, however, she has been having more difficulty falling asleep at night, mostly because she is worrying about her schoolwork. She also seems to crash on some weekends, as she is so tired from the long week.

The Numbers

- **Average hours of sleep:** 10 to 11 hours
- **Range:** 8 to $12^{3}/_{4}$ hours

Developmental Issues and Sleep

Your child will continue to grow and change throughout childhood. These important changes will affect your child's sleep.

- **Thinking skills.** Although a six-year-old is clearly a very different animal from a twelve-year-old when it comes to thinking skills, school-aged children as a group are maturing rapidly. They are becoming capable of absorbing more information, understanding complicated concepts, and thinking more abstractly about ideas. Children at this age are true "sponges" when it comes to new information and are fascinated by the world around them, although they may not always be able to reliably sort out fiction from fact. This is also prime time for children to start learning about their bodies, how they work, and what keeps them healthy. Not only that, they may actually still *listen* to you at this age. So what better time to introduce your child to the scientific wonders of the world of sleep, and also to begin to build a foundation for a lifetime of healthy sleep habits? All of us— parents, teachers, health care providers—have a responsibility to let kids know how important sleep is for staying healthy and doing well in school. We should also provide them with the best possible information about getting good sleep.

- **More responsibility and control.** As they approach the preteen years, children begin to take on more responsibility for (and more control of) their behavior and their health. Parents begin to loosen the reins on how kids dress, what they eat, and, yes, what time they go to bed. But just when parents are less likely to set and enforce a bedtime, kids may need parents to step in and take charge even more. For one thing, it becomes increasingly critical for middle-schoolers to get enough sleep in order to do all the complicated things they need to do in their average day. Although middle-schoolers may somewhat appreciate the value of sleep (or at least know how cranky their friends are after a sleepover), they may not yet have the skills and maturity to turn off the TV and go to bed. They may also need grown-up help in managing their time in the evening so that they can get to bed at a reasonable hour. They may actually *like* the structure (though they'd never admit it!) of their parents telling them when to go to bed.

- **More activities.** In addition, sleep slips further and further down the priority list (and the family's "to do" list as well) as school-aged kids become more and more involved in academic, social, athletic, and family activities. Television, computers, video games, and the Internet all compete increasingly for sleep time. Parents' work and activity schedules spilling over into the evening hours may also conflict with time for sleep, by pushing the dinner hour and homework time later and later.

- **More worries.** Although we as parents like to think of our children as not having a care in the world at this age, the reality is that kids worry about all kinds of things. They worry about being popular, about getting along with their friends, about doing well in school, and about something happening to themselves or to their parents. And worrying, especially when it's time for bed, is not very compatible with the relaxed state of mind needed to fall asleep. So if your school-aged child or middle-schooler is having trouble falling asleep all of a sudden, find out what's on her mind.

Common Sleep Issues

Although the general wisdom has always been that sleep problems are rare in school-aged children, sleep problems are much more common in this age group than you think. For example, about a third of parents of four- to ten-year-olds report at least one sleep problem; about a quarter fight bedtime, and one in ten have major problems falling asleep. It also seems that sleep problems don't always just go away as children get older.

- **Blissful ignorance.** The numbers given above might actually underestimate the problem. That is because they are based on parent reports, and many parents are actually *unaware* of their child's sleep concerns, especially at this age. One study found that children who were old enough to be somewhat reliable reporters (second grade and up) stated that they had significantly more difficulty falling asleep and more night wakings than their parents reported. These kids may not have complained to their parents (although they did to the researcher) about their sleep problems. It definitely pays to ask.
- **Daytime sleepiness.** From a purely physiologic standpoint, school-aged children are about the most alert human beings on earth. That means they usually have an almost nonexistent tendency to fall asleep during the day. It also means that when they *are* falling asleep in class, in the car, or in front of the TV on a regular basis, *something is wrong!* Assume, until proven otherwise, that if this is happening

to your child, it means he is not getting enough sleep, the sleep he is getting is not good, or both. You can also assume that falling asleep is just the tip of the sleepiness iceberg. If your child is actually dozing off in class, then much of the rest of the time when he's not asleep, he's on the edge of it. And that's not a good place to be. Unfortunately, this situation is also not that uncommon. In fact, in the study described above of four- to ten-year-olds, their teachers who were surveyed reported that one in ten of their students (kindergarten through fourth grade) was significantly sleepy at school.

LACK OF SLEEP

Lack of sleep affects *mood*. A sleepy child is more:

- irritable
- cranky
- moody
- whiny

Lack of sleep affects *learning*. A sleepy child has:

- a shorter attention span
- difficulty focusing
- a harder time remembering things
- difficulty solving problems

Lack of sleep affects *behavior*. A sleepy child is more likely to:

- misbehave
- be aggresive
- be hyperactive
- be uncooperative

Lack of sleep affects *health* in that it:

- lowers immune function (child is more likely to get colds, flu)
- increases accidental injuries
- affects growth hormone secretion

- **Circadian preference.** Children begin to show what's called their *circadian preference* at about this age. Meaning that when it comes to when they prefer to go to sleep at night and get up in the morning, some of them (and us) are clearly "night owls." Some are "morning larks." And others are somewhere between the two. This circadian preference is an important part of a child's sleep personality and affects how well he functions at certain times of the day. For example, some kids are more alert and on target in the morning, while others hit their stride in the afternoon or evening. What's important is having a sense of your child's "feeling best" times of the day and, when possible, schedule activities around those (like doing homework in the afternoon right after school versus later in the evening, or the other way around).

  Circadian preference can also have an impact on bedtime behavior. If your child prefers a later bedtime and morning wake-up time, he may have difficulty falling asleep. He may also protest about going to bed if his bedtime is a lot earlier than the time that his internal clock is set. However, in contrast to children who resist bedtime because they are defiant or have trouble accepting limits, children who are "night owls" will fall asleep easily and quickly at a later bedtime. Allowing your child to sleep on a schedule he selects himself for several days (like during a school vacation) may help you figure out your child's circadian preference and work with it.

- **Growing up fast.** As children reach the middle-school years, they may begin to show some of the sleep changes that go along with puberty and life as a teenager. If your middle-school child is an early maturer (lucky you!), you might want to take a peek at chapter 18 on adolescent sleep to see what lies ahead!

Common Sleep Problems

As mentioned above, sleep problems are common throughout the school years.

- **Bad sleep habits.** Poor sleep habits commonly develop during the school years. With more access to things like caffeine and television, as well as homework and an abundance of activities to fill

your child's day, good sleep habits often get lost in the shuffle. To
be sure your child gets the sleep that she needs, see chapter 6.

- **Not getting enough sleep.** Not getting enough sleep is surprisingly
  common in school-aged children. Be sure your child's schedule
  allows for enough hours of sleep at night.

- **Sleepwalking and sleep terrors.** Although these two sleep issues
  peak during the preschool years, school-aged children often continue to walk in their sleep and have sleep terrors. For most children, the frequency of these events decreases as they get older,
  usually disappearing after puberty. (See chapter 12 for more information on these two sleep problems.)

- **Obstructive sleep apnea.** Sleep apnea also peaks during the preschool years, but many school-aged children have sleep apnea,
  especially in the early elementary-school years. If you have concerns about your child's snoring or having breathing issues when
  he is sleeping, see chapter 13.

- **Restless legs syndrome/Periodic limb movement disorder.** It's still
  unclear at what age these two sleep disorders are most likely to
  emerge, but many adults who have them report that their symptoms started in childhood. Both of these sleep disorders involve leg
  symptoms, and cause problems either falling asleep or during sleep
  (see chapter 14).

Adolescents (12 to 18 years)

*Michael is fifteen, and like most fifteen-year-olds he stays up late at night, well
past the time his parents go to bed. It is always a fight on school mornings to get
him out of bed. If he doesn't have anything scheduled, he'll sleep until at least
noon on weekends. Michael is a very good student, but he has recently been
zoning out in school because he's so tired.*

The Numbers

- **Hours of sleep:** 9 to $9\frac{1}{2}$ hours needed on average; most teens get 7
  to $7\frac{1}{4}$ hours.
- **Range:** $6\frac{1}{2}$ to 10 hours

Developmental Issues and Sleep

Your son or daughter is no longer a child, but not yet an adult either (in so many ways!). Sleep is similar. Your child still needs the sleep of a younger child, but as his body matures, he's moving to a more adultlike schedule. Because there are so many issues surrounding sleep during adolescence, a full chapter on this topic is provided in chapter 18. Highlights of these issues are provided here.

- **Puberty.** In addition to all the other changes that occur at puberty, there is a shift in an adolescent's internal clock of about two hours. This shift results in your teenager going to bed about two hours later and waking up about two hours later.
- **Sleep need.** At the same time, though, adolescents still need a lot of sleep at night, about 9 to $9\frac{1}{4}$ hours per night. However, teens only get about 7 to $7\frac{1}{2}$ hours of sleep at night. This results in most teens being chronically sleep deprived.
- **Decreased daytime alertness.** In addition to the above changes in sleep, teenagers experience more sleepiness during the day. We are not totally sure why this happens, but it may be related to all the changes going in on in their bodies.

Common Sleep Issues

As mentioned, there are a plethora of sleep issues during the adolescent years. A complete discussion is provided in chapter 18.

- **Life's demands.** School and social demands, such as homework, after-school jobs, and social activities, often lead to adolescents going to bed later at night.
- **Weekdays versus weekends.** Teens are notorious for going to bed much later and sleeping until well past noon on weekends. The same thing often happens on school vacations and during the summer.
- **Early high-school start times.** At the same that a teen's internal clock shifts later, high schools typically start very early in the morning, usually earlier than middle schools start. Most teens have

not gotten the sleep that they need when it's time to get up for school.

- **Benign neglect.** Although many parents of teenagers relinquish control over their teen's bedtime, the reality is that they may need to be even more vigilant about sleep at this age. (See chapter 18 for suggestions on how to do this.)
- **High achievers.** Teens who are high achievers and involved in many extracurricular activities are particularly at risk for not getting enough sleep.

SLEEPY TEENS

Adolescents in the United States, as a group, are chronically sleep deprived. Many teens function for a good part of the day in the "twilight zone," which is a level of sleepiness equivalent to that found in people with narcolepsy!

Therefore, parents need to monitor their child's sleep and help their teenager schedule enough time in the day to get a good night's sleep.

Chronically not getting enough sleep may result in:

- poor performance in school.

- use of substances such as caffeine and stimulant medications to try to stay awake.

- increased risk-taking behaviors (such as use of alcohol and illicit drugs), injuries and motor vehicle crashes.

Common Sleep Problems

- **Not getting enough sleep.** As mentioned, adolescents are notorious for not getting enough sleep. Most teenagers are basically "walking zombies" from being chronically sleep deprived and spend a good deal of their waking hours pretty much in a daze.
- **Poor sleep habits.** Caffeine use, increased time on the computer and playing video games, and shifting sleep schedules on weekends all increase during the teen years.

- **Delayed sleep phase syndrome.** Delayed sleep phase syndrome peaks during the teen years. This sleep disorder involves an internal clock that is shifted later compared to the rest of society. Rather than having a clock set to sleep from 11:00 PM TO 8:00 AM, these teenagers' internal clocks are set closer to something like a bedtime of 3:00 AM and a wake time of 11:00 AM. As you can imagine, this leads to major problems, including chronic tardiness and even missing school. (See chapter 15 for more information on delayed sleep phase syndrome.)
- **Insomnia.** During the teenage years, some adolescents begin to have difficulty falling asleep at bedtime. For most, this is related to a delayed sleep phase, but some teenagers do develop insomnia in the sense that they have problems falling asleep at any bedtime. (Chapter 11 provides information on insomnia and how to deal with it.)
- **Restless legs syndrome/Periodic limb movement disorder.** These two sleep disorders cause problems either falling asleep or during sleep. Restless legs syndrome is an uncomfortable sensation in the legs that primarily occurs at bedtime. Periodic limb movement disorder involves limb movements that disrupt sleep (see chapter 14).
- **Narcolepsy.** Although a rare disorder, narcolepsy typically develops during adolescence. The hallmark of this disorder is severe daytime sleepiness (see chapter 16).

ASLEEP AT THE WHEEL

Older adolescent boys are among the highest risk group for drowsy-driving accidents. The most common drowsy-driving accident involves a single vehicle with a single driver who drives off the road late at night or in the middle of the afternoon. All adolescents with insufficient sleep are at risk, especially when a beer or two, marijuana, and relatively limited driving experience compound lack of sleep.

4

Bedtime Stories:
Common Myths about Kids and Sleep

One of the biggest challenges faced by those of us who specialize in solving children's sleep problems is dealing with all the misinformation that is out there. Lots of well-intentioned parents get advice from equally well-meaning friends, grandparents, and other parents about their child's sleep. Some of this advice is good information, and some of it is *just plain wrong*. New research is coming out every day that challenges a lot of our old beliefs and misconceptions about how and why we sleep. So sometimes, when you actually look at the facts, things that have always seemed like common sense about sleep turn out to be not so sensible after all. And unfortunately, not all of the information on TV, the Internet, or in books or magazines is correct, either. But you as a parent can help make sense of all this. Do your homework. Learn the facts. And make sure the sleep facts you are hearing or reading are accurate by going to the best and most reliable information sources available (see appendix B). Also, be proactive. Ask your child's pediatrician for information about healthy sleep habits and how to prevent sleep problems from happening in the first place. And don't hesitate to ask your doctor questions if you have specific concerns about your child's sleep.

Listed below are some of the more common myths we hear from parents (and from kids) about sleep, many of which you have probably heard (and perhaps believe) yourself. Each is followed by some of the reasons why they're fiction and not fact, and what the *real* skinny is about sleep.

Myth: *There are some children who just don't need very much sleep.*

Fact: Research has shown that the average adult needs *at least* eight hours of sleep to be at his or her best. There do appear to be some individual differences, in that some people seem to need slightly more or less than the eight-hour average (but no one, not even Martha Stewart, needs just four hours). However, most adults who think they need less sleep are kidding themselves. This is because we all tend to underestimate how sleepy we are and how a lack of adequate sleep affects us, and to overestimate how much we can actually compensate for lack of sleep.

Although there has been less research looking at sleep needs in children, we do know that the vast majority of children and adolescents need a certain amount of sleep, within a range that is based on their age. Sure, your child might get by in the short run with less, just as he could probably survive on a diet of cheeseburgers and fries, but why take the risk of shortchanging his ability to learn and function at his best? Don't make the mistake of assuming that the amount of sleep your child typically *gets* is the same as the amount of sleep he *needs*. Look for clues; a well-rested child wakes up by herself in the morning in a good mood and ready to face the day; doesn't nap (past the age of five or so), fall asleep in the car, or sleep in on weekends; and is alert and attentive throughout the day. Don't settle for less!

Myth: *Kids can "learn" not to need as much sleep.*

Fact: The amount of sleep that each of us needs is hard-wired into our genes and can't be changed. As much as we would all like to think we can fool Mother Nature, human beings do not "adapt" or "learn" to get less sleep with practice. Kids (especially teens) can learn to deal with being sleep deprived by cutting corners or cutting back on the amount of work they try to do, but that is not always an option. To a certain extent, you can also overcome (but only temporarily) the effects of sleep deprivation by putting in more effort. However, the end result is not the same as getting enough sleep.

RECOMMENDED TOTAL HOURS OF SLEEP		
AGE GROUP	**AGE**	**RECOMMENDED HOURS**
Infants	2 months to 12 months	14–15 hours
Toddlers	12 months to 3 years	12–14 hours
Preschoolers	3 years to 6 years	11–13 hours
School-aged	6 years to 12 years	10–11 hours
Adolescents	12 years to 18 years	8.5–9.5 hours

Myth: *It might make you grumpy, but not getting enough sleep doesn't really hurt you in the long run.*

Fact: There is more and more scientific evidence to suggest that, over time, not getting enough sleep or getting poor quality sleep could have devastating consequences for your child's mental and physical health. We know that children with certain sleep disorders that disrupt sleep, such as obstructive sleep apnea, have more learning, attention, and behavior problems and do less well in school. These children may also develop growth problems and, in severe cases, may end up with cardiovascular (heart and blood pressure) problems as well. Poor sleep has been linked to problems with the immune system, which can lead to less resistance to infections. In addition, children who get less sleep have been shown to have more accidental injuries. In adults, studies suggest that inadequate sleep may be associated with a greater risk of obesity and even with higher mortality rates. Just about every system in the body you can name can be negatively affected by sleep loss.

Myth: *Sleeping late on the weekends will make up for lost sleep during the week.*

Fact: Getting less than the amount of sleep that you need night after night accumulates over time and starts to create what we call a "sleep debt." And like all debts, eventually it needs to be paid off. The problem with waiting until the weekend to meet these sleep obligations is that in the meantime, your child is paying the price by being less alert, moodier, thinking slower, and having less motivation, just when she needs to be at her sharpest.

Sleeping in on weekends also makes it that much more difficult to get back on a weekday sleep schedule on Monday morning. Imagine the jet lag a person experiences when traveling back and forth from the East Coast to the West Coast every weekend. That's what happens to your child's internal clock when he goes to bed and gets up three or four hours later on Friday and Saturday night and then tries to fall asleep at a normal school bedtime on Sunday.

Myth: *Drinking caffeinated sodas (or coffee) can make up for lost sleep.*

Fact: These substances and other stimulants may temporarily increase your alertness level by acting on certain chemicals in the brain (neurotransmitters) that regulate sleep. *But they are not a substitute for sleep.* Neither is just closing your eyes or "resting." That's because both your body and brain renew and revitalize themselves while you sleep, and in order for this process to happen, you have to go through all the normal stages of sleep. So the only thing that replaces sleep is sleep.

Myth: *A boring teacher (warm room, full stomach, etc.) can put kids to sleep.*

Fact: If your child is getting enough sleep on a regular basis, there is no teacher (math book, reading assignment) in the world boring enough to make him fall asleep in class. There are basically two things that make people sleepy: not getting *enough* sleep, and not getting *good quality* sleep. The environment a person is in (the room temperature, the light level) may unmask underlying sleepiness but *does not cause it!* So if your child (especially your school-aged child) is dozing off in class (in the car, watching TV), don't ignore it or chalk it up to bad teachers . . . investigate!

Myth: *Sleeping more makes kids feel more tired.*

Fact: One of the ways that the body tries to make up for not getting enough sleep is to increase the amount of deep sleep (also called *slow wave*). Slow wave sleep is believed to be the most restorative or restful type (or stage) of sleep. It is also particularly important in childhood, because it is the stage of sleep during which most growth hormone is released in the body. The more sleep deprived someone is, the greater the percentage of deep sleep he has as the body tries to recover from the effects of sleep loss. If a person is awakened during slow wave sleep, she is likely to be very groggy, confused, and disoriented, a condition known as *sleep inertia*. Parents and kids sometimes think this grogginess means that they are sleeping too much when, in fact, their bodies are just trying their hardest to make up for lost sleep.

Myth: *The worst part of kids' snoring is how annoying it is to everyone else.*

Fact: In fact, snoring can be a sign of a serious sleep problem called *obstructive sleep apnea,* or OSA (see chapter 13). Once thought to occur mostly in adults, we now know that sleep apnea affects at least 1 percent of all children and a greater percent of certain higher-risk groups. These include children with large tonsils, children who are overweight and obese, those with allergies/asthma, and children with Down syndrome. About 10 percent of all children snore regularly, and it is estimated that about one in ten of these children have OSA. This sleep disorder can lead to serious medical consequences as well as learning and behavior problems. OSA is also an important cause of symptoms of ADHD. Don't ignore snoring in your child or adolescent; make sure to inform your child's doctor!

Myth: *Teenagers can "pull an all-nighter" to study and still be ready for the big test in the morning.*

Fact: Teenagers would actually be much better off studying less and getting a good night's sleep. Research clearly shows that the ability to concentrate and learn new information, as well as to work efficiently, falls off sharply after being awake for fifteen or sixteen hours in a row, and continues to bottom out the longer you stay up. And if the big test is at 8:00 AM, the problem is even worse. That's because that time of day is also typically a low energy point in the body's normal twenty-four-hour circadian rhythm (especially in teenagers). Finally, there have been fascinating studies showing the importance of sleep in learning and memory. One study took a group of students and had them all learn the same material on day one. That night the students either got a full night's sleep or pulled an all-nighter. One week later they tested the students. Those who slept the night after learning the material did much better on the test than those who hadn't slept. Remember, this was one week later! Thus, getting sleep after learning information seems important for memory consolidation. So pulling an all-nighter is not a good recipe for making the grade.

Myth: *Teenagers who want to sleep late in the morning are just plain lazy.*

Fact: Scientific evidence clearly shows that puberty is associated with more than just raging hormones. There are dramatic changes in sleep that occur with puberty as well. One of the most important sleep developments is a shift in the natural biological sleep and wake schedule to a later bedtime and wake time. In other words, teenagers just can't fall asleep as early and wake as early as they did in elementary and middle school, because their internal clocks have shifted. At the same time, teens still really need nine hours of sleep a night to be well rested. So the late bedtimes dictated by biology and the early wake-up times enforced by school systems just don't cut it.

Myth: *It's elderly drivers, not teenage drivers, who are the ones falling asleep at the wheel. After all, teenagers can tell when they're too tired to drive safely!*

Myth: *And if you do get drowsy while driving, you can always splash some cold water on your face (turn up the radio, get some fresh air) and be on your way.*

Facts: Believing these common myths can literally have deadly consequences. Studies show that the highest risk group for drowsy-driving crashes is sixteen-to-thirty-year-olds, especially young men. Not only are they less experienced and riskier drivers, they are more likely to be sleep deprived. They are also more likely to combine sleepiness with alcohol, marijuana, or other drugs, which makes the risk of a drowsy-driving accident even higher.

All of us, not just teenagers, tend to underestimate our level of sleepiness and overestimate our ability to overcome the effects of sleepiness. Furthermore, the sleepier someone is, the less able he is to appreciate it. Worst of all, it is possible for your brain to fall asleep for several seconds *(microsleep)* without you even realizing it. In one study of sleep-deprived medical residents, for example, they reported being "awake" three-quarters of the time that they actually were asleep!

Finally, almost none of the things we all do to fight off sleepiness while driving (turn on the radio, pinch ourselves, chew gum) work for more than a few minutes. The best way to handle drowsy driving is to prevent it in the first place by getting enough sleep or being smart enough not to drive if you are sleepy (take a cab, find a friend who can give you a lift home). If all else fails, pull over, get off the road, and get to somewhere safe where you can sleep.

PART TWO: **SLEEP STRATEGIES**

5

Sleep Stealers: What May Be Robbing Your Child of a Good Night's Sleep

John is twelve years old. He's a typical middle-schooler, and takes karate lessons once a week and on Saturdays, plays soccer in a local league, and is in the church choir. He usually drinks Mountain Dew or Coke at lunch and dinner. His parents try to watch what he eats, as he has a tendency to be a bit overweight. Most nights after completing his homework, he heads up to his room. There he watches television, plays computer games, and instant messages his friends until it's time to go to bed.

John is a fairly typical twelve-year-old, one whose life is full of sleep-stealers that neither he nor his parents are aware of. Caffeine, multiple after-school activities, a tendency to be overweight, and a room full of electronics are all par for the course these days. But all of these things can rob your child of a good night's sleep. These top four common sleep-stealers are discussed here, as well as what you can do to help your child get the sleep that he needs.

The Electronic Sandman

One of the biggest and baddest boogeymen in and out of the bedroom that you as a parent face is the wonderful world of electronic media. After all, what child, when tempted by twenty-four-hour cable networks or the seductive flickering glare of the computer screen, would actually choose to *go to bed?* What teenager would pass up the opportunity to instant message the object of a budding romance until midnight every night just to get some shut-eye, however badly needed? And for that matter, what adult can resist "just one more" segment of Letterman or Leno before he or she turns in for the night?

A survey of sleep and television viewing in children we conducted about eight years ago in a largely middle-class New England suburb found that 25 percent of kindergarten through fourth-graders had television sets in their bedroom. The Kaiser Family Foundation in 2000 reported that one-third of two-to-seven-year-olds and two-thirds of eight-to-eighteen-year-olds already have a television in their bedroom. And the most recent data from 2004 shows that this number is continuing to grow; a National Sleep Foundation poll found that 30 percent of preschoolers and 43 percent of school-aged children have a television in their bedroom. What's more, the National Institute on Media and the Family reported that children with a television in their bedroom are likely to spend an additional five and a half hours a week watching it. That's about forty-five minutes a day that could be better spent reading, playing outside, or *sleeping.*

The American Academy of Pediatrics recommends that children's bedrooms be "media-free zones." That means no computer, video games, PlayStation, Game Boy, and no television set. Period. If you have not yet put a television in your child's room, don't! If you have already gone down that slippery slope, think very seriously about removing it. This is the kind of advice that, understandably, makes parents cringe, and there is no way we are pretending that this is an easy task. But let's review how TV can become a "sleep stealer" and why it just might be worth braving the screams of protest you are likely to encounter:

- **It can lead to sleep problems.** Children who watch a lot of television, watch television as part of their bedtime routine, and especially children who have a television in their room are more likely to have sleep problems. These include difficulty falling asleep, anxiety at bedtime, and night wakings. These children are also more likely to get less sleep than they need. Granted, this is only an association and does not prove cause and effect. That is, there might be a bit of a chicken-and-egg phenomenon going on here. It may be that children who have problems falling asleep to begin with might be more likely to watch TV to "help" them fall asleep. However, there are also a number of important reasons why trying to use the background noise and soft glow of a TV to fall asleep are a bad idea at best.

- **It's a stimulating activity.** Television watching (and this applies equally or more to video games and computer games) is much more likely to wake kids up than to put them to sleep. In other words, watching TV is counterproductive to achieving the state of relaxation that we all need in order to fall asleep. Think about it. Television programming is all about "what's coming up next." The whole point is to try to hook the viewer into watching one more segment, one more episode, one more show. You, as an adult, might be able to ignore that message, but most kids can't.

- **It's easy to become dependent.** If you need the television on to fall asleep at bedtime, you're much more likely to need it to fall back asleep if you wake up during the night. This is a basic principle of what is known as "conditioning." For example, if you always wear the same red sweater whenever you give an important presentation, then you are likely to feel somewhat panicked if it's not available the next time around. And since night wakings in kids are common, it's easy to create a situation in which they "need" the television on at 3:00 AM to get back to sleep. We can't tell you how many kids we see in our sleep clinic who watch television at all hours of the night, often completely unbeknownst to their unsuspecting parents.

- **It's anti-sleep.** There may be some biological reasons why television watching might be "anti-sleep." Noise and particularly light, even low levels of light, can make falling asleep more difficult. Remember, light prevents the brain from turning on the production of the hormone melatonin, which in turn is absolutely critical to turning on sleep. The bottom line is that bedrooms should be for quiet activities like reading, listening to music, daydreaming, and above all, sleeping.

- **It's easy to lose control.** To quote Joan Anderson, author of *Getting Unplugged and Breaking the TV Habit,* "TV is not a member of the family; it's a stranger. Would you let a stranger into your child's bedroom?" No matter what you think and how well-intentioned you are as a parent, once you've put that television in your child's bedroom, you've lost a lot of control over what, when, why, and how much TV your child watches. According to a 1999 study by the National Institute on Media and the Family, while 81 percent of parents are concerned about the amount of violence their children see in movies on television, only 58 percent have rules about television viewing. You may reassure yourself that you have clear rules about television viewing in your household, but by putting a television in your child's room, you've lost much of your ability to enforce those rules. Ditto for playing computer and video games.

- **It cuts down on family time.** A television set in each household member's bedroom may cut down on arguments about what to watch. But it also means you've basically eliminated TV viewing as a shared family activity. You lose precious moments of "family time." In addition, you lose the opportunity to interact with your kids about what's on the tube, to share opinions, to put what they're watching in perspective, to talk about what might be scary, and maybe to find out more about what they like and who they are as people.

- **It can lead to obesity.** Numerous studies have found a relationship between TV watching and obesity in kids. The more television children watch (and the more time spent playing video or computer games), the more inactive they are, and the more weight they are likely to gain. Not to mention the constant bombardment of television advertising aimed at getting kids to eat stuff that is high in sugar, high in fat, and low in nutritional value. And being overweight or obese, in addition to all the other bad health effects, can also affect your sleep (see pages 58–60).

- **It can affect your dreams.** What your child watches can affect her dreams. JoAnne Cantor's book, *"Mommy, I'm Scared": How TV and Movies Frighten Children and What We Can Do to Protect Them*, eloquently describes the negative effects that the vivid visual pictures on the television screen can have on children (and the same would certainly apply to computer-game graphics). As an adult, you can process and put into context the disturbing images you see on the nightly news or the latest crime drama, but your child may not be able to do the same and may incorporate those images into nightmares.

WHAT A PARENT CAN DO

- **Don't put a television set in your child's bedroom.** If there is one in there already, take it out. After all, having a television in your room is *not* a God-given unalienable childhood right.

- **Create a homework zone.** If possible, set up a quiet area of the house for studying that is free from distractions but accessible enough to keep an eye on things. Put the computer there instead of in the bedroom.

- **Use modern technology to your advantage.** If all else fails, (and granted, this does mean that you finally have to learn to program the VCR) you can always tape (or TiVo) the darn show and watch it the next day. Contrary to what your child may claim, this is *not* borderline child abuse, and may even enable you to watch it together (come on, one episode of *The OC* won't kill you).

- **Don't make TV part of the bedtime routine.** Make the last thing your child remembers as she slips into dreamland the soothing sound of *your* voice reading the next chapter of Harry Potter, instead of the latest episode of some sitcom.

- **Step up to the plate.** Finally (and this is painful), you may want to consider *taking the TV out of your bedroom as well,* for many of the same reasons cited above. Not for nothing, this is a golden opportunity to be a terrific role model. And as a bonus, you just might get a better night's sleep yourself.

Mountain Dew to Starbucks: The Caffeine Connection

It's everywhere—in the coffee and cocoa we sip, the chocolate bars we munch, the soda we gulp, and in the tea we drink. It's there in huge amounts in those cleverly named "energy" beverages that are specifically marketed for kids and teens: Jolt, Red Bull, Monster, and Buzz Water. It's the main ingredient in Bawls, a carbonated drink sold over the Internet that boasts that it's the most highly caffeinated beverage on the market and that it allows you to stay up all night and play computer games ("the perfect drink to make sure you don't lag behind"). Caffeine is the most commonly used drug in America (and in the world).

Yes, that's right, *drug*. Caffeine and its "sister" chemicals, theophylline and theobromine (which are also found in varying amounts in beverages like coffee, tea, colas, etc.), are central nervous system stimulants. This means they give you a "buzz" or a sense of increased alertness (theobromine is considerably weaker than caffeine and theophylline, having about one-tenth the stimulating effect of either). While theophylline and theobromine relax smooth muscle (that's how theophylline works as an asthma drug), they and caffeine are also cardiac stimulants (they increase your heart rate). They are also diuretics, which means they make your body produce more urine. All of these effects are related to the fact that caffeine inhibits a specific enzyme in the body (cyclic AMP phosphodiesterase, in case you wanted to know) that controls many body functions.

Caffeine is also addictive, in the sense that people develop a physical dependence upon it and have withdrawal symptoms if they stop. If you feel like you just can't function without it and need to drink (or take) something with caffeine every day, then you are addicted to caffeine.

CAFFEINE		
PRODUCT	SERVING SIZE	CAFFEINE CONTENT (mg)
SODAS		
Coca-Cola	8 oz.	23
Diet Coke	8 oz.	31
Diet Pepsi	8 oz.	24
Pepsi	8 oz.	25
Dr. Pepper/Diet Dr. Pepper	8 oz.	28
Mountain Dew/Diet Mountain Dew	8 oz.	47
Sunkist	8 oz.	28

PRODUCT	SERVING SIZE	CAFFEINE CONTENT (mg)
"CAFFEINE" DRINKS		
Bawls	10 oz.	80
Buzz Water	12 oz.	200
Jolt	12 oz.	70
Red Bull	11 oz.	80
COFFEE		
Arizona Blue Luna Iced Coffees	8 oz.	40–50
Cappuccino	6 oz.	35
Coffee, decaf	8 oz.	5
Starbucks Coffee, grande	16 oz.	550
Starbucks Coffee, tall	12 oz.	375
TEA		
Iced Tea	8 oz.	25
Mistic Teas	8 oz.	17
Snapple iced tea (all kinds)	8 oz.	21
OTHER		
Baker's chocolate	1 oz.	26
Chocolate milk	8 oz.	5
Coffee ice cream	8 oz.	58
Dark chocolate, semi-sweet	1 oz.	20
MEDICATIONS		
Anacin	2 tablets	65
Dexatrim	1 tablet	200
Excedrin, max. strength	2 tablets	130
Midol	1 tablets	32
No-Doz, max. strength; Vivarin	1 tablet	200
No-Doz, regular strength	1 tablet	100

The Good (sort of) News: The potential benefits of caffeine are that it delays (but does not eliminate!) fatigue and provides a temporary "boost of energy." (All information about caffeine also applies to theophylline and theobromine as well.) Caffeine starts to work as soon as fifteen minutes after it is consumed. Its effects last about three to four hours. It's often used by people (particularly by college students, truck drivers, and shift workers) to help them stay awake longer. Caffeine does work fairly well for a short time for this purpose, but it is not a substitute for sleep. Caffeine may help you stay awake and alert enough to study, but it will not improve your performance on an exam the next day if you have not gotten enough sleep. Also, importantly, caffeine does not counteract the effects of alcohol. In other words, coffee does not make a drunk person sober or fit to drive.

CAFFEINE IS NOT A SUBSTITUTE FOR SLEEP!

One of the other touted benefits of caffeine is weight loss. Because it increases the metabolism of fatty acids, it has been used for years by runners and dieters. Caffeine is not an appetite suppressant, however, so its real usefulness as a diet aid is questionable. Despite that, over-the-counter diet aids, such as Dexatrim, typically have 200 milligrams of caffeine. You should be aware that herbal supplements for weight loss often contain substantial levels of caffeine as well. They may also contain guarana or ephedra (ma huang)—other nervous system stimulants.

And the Bad News: No matter what the potential benefits of caffeine may be, there's also a price to pay. First, once it is in the body, caffeine will stay around for hours. It takes about six hours for one-half of the caffeine to be eliminated from your body, but it can last much longer in some folks (like the elderly). Also, some people are clearly more sensitive to the effects of caffeine than others; some of this depends on how big you are and how much you weigh. Which is why caffeine, particularly later in the day, so often causes difficulty falling asleep and disrupts sleep.

Second, once you've become dependent on caffeine, stopping it is a big problem. Typical withdrawal symptoms associated with caffeine are headache, fatigue, and muscle pain. This headache, well known among coffee drinkers, usually lasts from one to five days. Often people who are reducing their caffeine intake, in addition to having a headache, are irritable, nervous, jumpy, and less able to concentrate. In some cases they get nauseous and vomit. These symptoms can occur as soon as twenty-four hours after the last dose of caffeine.

Other potential risks associated with caffeine include possible effects on the fetus in pregnant women. Although the effects in humans remain controversial, it is known that caffeine causes malformations in rats when ingested at extremely high rates. In any case, most doctors suggest that pregnant women avoid caffeine or at least consume it in moderation. In addition, theobromine is also highly toxic to dogs, and "chocolate poisoning" can be fatal. A few M&Ms won't hurt a dog, but a pound of chocolate could do a lot of damage. On the other hand, the suggested links between caffeine and cancer, heart disease (although it may cause temporary increases in blood pressure in sensitive people), osteoporosis, and breast (fibrocystic) disease have, for the most part, not been supported by research.

Coffee Talk: *Coffee,* probably the best-known source of caffeine, contains mostly caffeine and some theophylline. But all coffee is certainly not created equal when it comes to creating a buzz. For example, the amount of caffeine in dark roast coffees and espresso (because it uses significantly more ground coffee than regular drip coffee and is prepared using pressurized water, resulting in a higher percentage of caffeine) is generally higher. A cup of strongly brewed coffee (or tea) has more caffeine than a weakly brewed cup. The caffeine content of some popular brews is listed on page 51.

Tea, which many people think has a lot less in the way of caffeine effects, actually does contain theophylline and theobromine, which can have stimulating effects similar to caffeine (herbal tea that is specifically labeled "caffeine-free" does not). Similarly, although the amount of caffeine in *cocoa* is relatively small, its theobromine content (about seven times greater than caffeine) clearly makes it "stimulating" as well.

For the average teenager, however, other sources of caffeine are probably both more important and more socially acceptable (and also more likely to be in the average high-school vending machine) than coffee or tea. The caffeine content of some of the most popular "youth beverages" are provided on page 51. For parents who think of caffeine only when it comes to colas, some of these may be a surprise. There are also lots of other beverages listed that many parents may not even be aware of because such beverages enjoy a more "underground" distribution. For example, Thinkgeek.com ("over 441,466,395 milligrams of caffeine served by ThinkGeek to its loyal fans since 1999. Wowzers!") is just one of a number of popular Web sites that advertise many kinds of "super-caffeinated" beverages and syrups. Some carry the highly suspect endorsement of being "natural stimulants" (for "people from all walks of life who enjoy the clean, crisp taste of guarana along with a powerful rush of caffeine"). Perhaps more disturbingly, Thinkgeek also features a wide assortment of caffeine gum, caffeine candy, and caffeine mints (Black Black gum and candy, Bawls mints, Jolt gum, Buzz Bites Chocolate Chews, Penguin mints and gums), and caffeine pills ("pocket size caffeine delivery vehicles"). Are we the only ones that find it deeply disturbing that the Leaders of Tomorrow seem to need so badly to drug themselves to stay awake today?

Finally, you should be aware that many over-the-counter medications advertised for other purposes also contain substantial amounts of caffeine. Products like Umph Energy Tablets, Enerjets, No-Doz Maximum Strength Caplets, and Vivarin are pretty clearly designed specifically for the three-o'clock-in-the-morning crowd. But the caffeine content in Anacin, Midol, and Dristan, for example, might not be so obvious. The real problem here is that many unsuspecting folks (including perhaps your kids) are getting caffeine from multiple sources at the same time.

The other hard fact of modern life is that prescription stimulants (such as Ritalin, Dexedrine, Concerta, and Adderall) are becoming more and more available as "street drugs." Most kids use them not so much to get high as to stay awake. It's quite easy for any high-school student to "score" some stimulant medication from a friend with ADHD (and, unfortunately, not impossible to get these drugs directly from an unsuspecting physician who is prescribing them for "attention problems" that are actually a direct result of lack of sleep). You need to be aware of the many ways a drug like caffeine can be and is (perfectly legally) consumed. You also need to be aware of the potential risks for your child, and aware that your middle-schooler or adolescent may be using stimulants during the day to counteract the effects of not getting enough sleep at night.

WHAT A PARENT CAN DO

- **Know the numbers.** Become familiar with the caffeine content of your child's favorite beverages. This is not typically listed in the ingredients, so you might have to play detective. The list we've given on page 50 will help get you started.
- **Keep track.** Figure out how much caffeine your child or teenager is consuming on a daily basis from all possible sources. Keep a careful record (and this will require your teenager's cooperation) of the amount and types of caffeine usually consumed in a typical week. You both may be surprised at how high the amounts are and where it's coming from (remember, 300 mg per day, the rough equivalent of three cups of coffee or three cans of Jolt cola, is considered "moderate" caffeine use).
- **Ask questions.** If your teenager seems to be consuming large amounts of caffeine on a daily basis, you need to figure out why. Maybe she's using it to help herself stay awake in class because she's not getting the sleep she needs. Or maybe your son is downing Mountain Dews all evening so he can stay up and play computer games all night. Whatever the reason, tackling that may eliminate the need for the caffeine in the first place.
- **Cut down.** Once you know what you're dealing with, make a plan with your child to eliminate caffeine or at least reduce it. There is really no reason for anyone to use caffeine, but there is particularly no rationale for younger children to have anything that contains it. There are plenty of healthier alternatives out there, such as caffeine-free soda, juice, and water.
- **Go slow.** The process known as "caffeine fading" is one way of beating the caffeine-withdrawal blues. Although you can always go "cold turkey," a more gradual reduction avoids potentially nasty withdrawal symptoms (especially the headache) and also gets the body used to functioning without the drug. Depending on where your child or teen starts

---

out, reduce caffeine intake at a rate that feels comfortable. For example, cutting down at the rate of $1/2$ cup of coffee (soda, Red Bull, whatever) works for some, while reducing caffeine intake in slower steps (two to five cups of coffee per week) is a more tolerable pace for others.

- **Take a stand.** Find out what your child's school vending machines have in them in the way of drinks. Make a pitch to the school to eliminate any caffeinated beverages. That goes for the lunch line as well (a local boarding school in one of the authors' hometowns recently added Starbucks coffee to the cafeteria menu, supposedly for the faculty's benefit).
- **Walk the walk.** Maybe you don't really need that double-shot espresso to get your engine started in the morning. Perhaps you wouldn't feel quite so jittery or have quite as much of a headache by the end of the day if you cut down on your caffeine-of-choice. View this as yet another golden role model opportunity.

Too many activities and too little time (for sleep, that is)

It is almost a fact of life that kids these days are overscheduled, overcommitted, overextended, and, as a result overtired. As parents, we tend to consider this a given, a sad but inevitable part of raising children in our competitive modern society. We might consider the "cramming schools" that many teenagers in Japan attend after-hours on school nights (meaning after 10:00 PM), as part of the traditional preparation for college entrance exams, a bit excessive. But we are equally quick to defend the long hours of studying for SATs and Stanley Kaplan courses as part of the price of doing business (college admission business, that is). We rationalize our teenager spending six hours a day at an after-school job as being what all kids do to earn a little extra gas money. And we defend the evening karate class, hockey practice, music lesson, or the multitude of other extracurricular activities as necessary to make our kids "well rounded."

The problem is, they may turn out to be well rounded, but not well rested. Kids who spend more time in extracurricular activities and after-school jobs, at the expense of sleep time, simply do less well at all of the above. It should be clear by now that lack of sleep compromises many of the skills that make for academic success—attention, organization, creative thinking, and efficiency. It also erodes the motivation that kids have to do well in the first place. Furthermore, without some wind-down time in the evening, the expectation that kids can easily go from full-throttle, sixty-miles-an-hour-active to all-of-a-sudden-fast-asleep is not only unrealistic but may contribute to some serious difficulties in their ability to fall asleep.

WHAT A PARENT CAN DO

- **Make compromises when it comes to your child's extracurricular activities instead of when it comes to sleep.** There are no easy choices here, especially if the pressure to do more, study more, and work more comes from your teenager herself. But driven kids often have driven parents. So ask yourself if you might be giving a subconscious but nonetheless crystal-clear message to your child that (a) getting enough sleep is optional, (b) you would be willing to sacrifice short-term sleep deprivation for the possibility of long-term academic gains, and (c) after all, you don't get a lot of sleep and look how well you're doing, you can't really expect them to do anything different.

- **Limit after-school job hours.** Recently a proposal to delay the high-school start time in a neighboring community was defeated, not because the school committee was against it (they weren't) but because the *students themselves voted it down.* And what was the overwhelming reason for the nay vote? They all wanted to get to their after-school jobs at McDonald's, Stop and Shop, and the mall so that they could get in as many hours as possible. A good work ethic is one thing, and teens deserve to have the opportunity to make some disposable income, but not at the expense of their schoolwork and decidedly not at the expense of their health.

- **Talk to the coach about those late-evening practice sessions.** This may not get you anywhere and probably will not make you the world's most popular parent with the athletic department (or some really gung-ho soccer moms and hockey dads), but it's worth a try. Sometimes a schedule gets set up more for someone's convenience than because there was no other choice. A little well-placed prod (particularly if you can get other parents on your side) and some gentle reminders about the consequences of sleep deprivation on things important to athletic performance like agility, stamina, and motivation might do the trick. And the team might just reap the benefits of having better-rested and better-prepared athletes in the process.

Overweight and overtired: How those excess pounds might be costing your child a good night's sleep.

It is clear from almost any newspaper or magazine article you read these days that we are a nation of overeaters, and as a consequence have one of the highest rates of obesity in the world. Sadly, this epidemic has now hit our country's children as well. In the 1970s, 4 percent of children six to eleven years old were obese. In 1999–2000 the figure rose to 15 percent and has continued to climb. Today nearly 22 percent of *preschool* children in the United States are defined as overweight and 10 percent as obese. Certain racial and ethnic groups (Mexican Americans, non-Hispanic blacks) are at an even higher risk for obesity. Obesity in children and teenagers is associated not only with obesity in adulthood, but also with an increased risk for heart disease, diabetes, and high blood pressure later in life.

But what does weight have to do with sleep? Plenty, evidently. First, there are now a number of studies that suggest there is *a link between sleep loss and weight gain*. Some of these studies (in adults) have looked at how sleep deprivation changes the body's normal metabolism and hormone function, and the results are not good. Not getting enough sleep seems to affect not only how (in)efficiently you metabolize calories, but also how hungry you feel (by altering the level of a number of hormones—serotonin, leptin, perhaps others—in the body). Think about how many times you've tried to keep yourself awake at 2:00 AM by eating doughnuts or pizza. Or how you've used a "carb fix" as a pick-me-up when feeling drowsy in the middle of the day (maybe this does more to explain the typical ten-pound weight gain of the sleep-deprived college-freshman than the calorie content of dining hall food). This hormonal imbalance may eventually place people at greater risk for diabetes as well.

Other research has also found a negative relationship between weight and sleep in children (the less you sleep, the more likely you are to be obese). One study in Japan found a link in six- and seven-year-olds between obesity and later bedtimes and fewer hours of sleep. Children who got less than eight hours of sleep had an almost three times greater risk of being obese compared to children who got ten or more hours. In addition, some of these studies suggest this relationship may also go in the other direction. In other words, the risk of being obese decreases with each additional hour that your child sleeps! This may well be the single greatest argument you'll ever have in getting your teenage daughter to go to bed at a reasonable hour.

In addition, being overweight or obese can greatly increase your child's chances of having a serious sleep disorder. Obstructive sleep apnea (see chapter 13) is a breathing disorder that occurs during sleep and affects about 1–3 percent of children in the United States. It often leads to problems with attention, behavior, and academics. The most common cause in children is large tonsils and adenoids. In adults, though, sleep apnea is most often related to being overweight or obese (the best predictor of sleep apnea in adults is having a neck size of seventeen inches or above). Over the past ten years in our sleep clinic, we have clearly evaluated more and more overweight and obese children and teenagers for sleep apnea. In fact, about two-thirds of the children we diagnose with sleep apnea are overweight or obese.

Overall, the risk of sleep apnea in obese children is four to five times that of normal weight children. Yet fewer than 50 percent of pediatricians state that they ask questions about sleep problems "most of the time or often" in their obese patients. So it is very important that parents of overweight children be aware of this possible link with sleep apnea. You should also be aware of the most common symptoms of sleep apnea (loud snoring, breathing pauses, restless sleep, daytime tiredness), so that these can be brought to the attention of your child's doctor for further evaluation.

The combination of obesity and sleep apnea may also have greater consequences than either condition alone. As it has in adults, sleep apnea in obese children has been associated with insulin resistance, a condition that increases the risk of heart disease, high triglyceride levels, and diabetes later on. Studies also suggest that both obesity and sleep apnea in children are independently associated with a decreased quality of life (physical, emotional, social, academic functioning) and together may present an even greater challenge.

Finally, the relationship between sleep and obesity may involve other issues. For example, in obese adolescents decreased physical activity and more disturbed sleep go hand in hand. This suggests that one possible factor in adolescent obesity might be poor quality sleep. Obesity leads to daytime fatigue, which makes teens less likely to exercise, which eventually leads to more weight gain, and so on. As already mentioned, children who watch a lot of television and spend most of their time in sedentary activities are more likely to be overweight. They are also more likely to have sleep problems, which, in turn, may result in their being less active, gaining more weight, and then developing more sleep problems.

WHAT A PARENT CAN DO

- **Limit fatty foods and foods high in calories.** Junk the junk food. Discourage between-meal snacks.
- **Encourage outdoor and physical activity.** Schedule time for your child to be outdoors and to spend at least thirty minutes a day being physically active.
- **Limit television viewing, computer time, and video games.** Cut back on all the electronics!
- **Watch out for school lunches.** Often the biggest culprits in the high-calorie, high-fat sweepstakes are the school cafeteria and vending machines. You probably have some handle on what your kids eat at home, but much less control over what they eat when they're out of your sight. This requires some combination of teaching your kids about healthy food choices and making sure the bad choices they do have are as limited as possible.
- **Be aware of the sleep and weight connection.** If your child is overweight, look for signs of obstructive sleep apnea, and let your pediatrician know if you see any of them. Make sure that lack of sleep doesn't play a role in causing the weight problem. Keep track of when and under what circumstances your child is most likely to overeat, and note if these are times when he seems sleepy or tired.
- **Make healthy eating, like healthy sleep, an important priority for your whole family.**

6

Ten Steps (and a few additional suggestions) to a Good Night's Sleep

Although there is no "magic pathway" to a good night's sleep, the following steps will help your child or adolescent get the best sleep possible and ease the journey into the Land of Nod.

Step 1: Put Sleep at the Top of Your "To Do" List

Make sleep a family priority. In our 24/7 society, sleep tends to be at the bottom of the priority list, but it shouldn't be. Sleep can make all the difference in how we feel and act the next day. To keep up with the fast-paced lifestyle of most families, sleep is a major help, not a hindrance.

Step 2: Have a Consistent Sleep Schedule . . . and Keep Weekends the Same

Have your child wake up and go to bed at about the same time on school nights and non–school nights. Bedtime and wake time should not differ from one day to the next by more than an hour or so. In addition, don't let your child sleep in too much on weekends to catch up on sleep. This will make it hard for your child to fall asleep at bedtime that night. If your child sleeps in until noon on Sunday, there is no way that he'll be able to go to sleep at 10:00 PM that night for school the next day. He literally won't have been awake enough hours to feel sleepy. Shifting the sleep-wake schedule back and forth by two to four hours on weekends versus weekdays is basically equivalent to having jet lag once a week. Picture a child who lives in New York City having to travel to and from Los Angeles every weekend, and you'll have some idea of what we mean.

Step 3: Remember, It's a BED-room.

Your child's bedroom should be comfortable, quiet, and dark. A nightlight is fine, as completely dark rooms can be scary for some young children. Your child will sleep better in a room that is cool (less than 75 degrees). Also, if your child is young, avoid using the bedroom for time-out or as a punishment. You want your child to think of his bedroom as a haven, not a prison. On the other hand, bedrooms should not be the home equivalent of Toys R' Us or Dave and Buster's (see steps 4 and 5).

Step 4: Banish the Bedroom TV

Get the television set out of your child's bedroom. According to a recent poll by the National Sleep Foundation, 43 percent of school-aged children and 30 percent of preschoolers have a television in their bedroom. These children who have a television in their bedroom go to bed later and get significantly less sleep than their peers. These findings are consistent with many studies that have found that a television in the bedroom interferes with sleep. In addition, children and adolescents can easily develop the bad habit of "needing" the TV to fall asleep. It is also much more difficult to control your child's TV viewing if the set is in the bedroom.

Step 5: Pull the Plug

Not only should you remove your child's television from his bedroom, but remove all other electronics too. Fifth-graders are no longer reading by flashlight under the covers, instead they are instant messaging their friends. Teenagers are staying up late playing online fantasy games or surfing the Internet. Move the computer to another space, leave the Game Boy in the family room, and take out the telephone (although these days with cordless phones that is much harder to do).

Step 6: Get a Routine

Your child should have a twenty- to thirty-minute bedtime routine that is the same every night. The routine should include calm activities, such as reading a book or talking about the day, with the last part occurring in the room where your child sleeps. Although we think of a bedtime routine as something for young children, older children and adolescents need a relaxing bedtime routine too.

In addition, the hour before bed should be a quiet or wind-down time. Your child should not get involved in high-energy activities, such as rough play or playing outside, or stimulating activities, such as playing computer games. Relaxing, calm, enjoyable activities like reading a book or listening to calm music will help your child's body and mind slow down enough to let him get to sleep.

In addition, your child should not go to bed hungry. A light snack (such as milk and cookies) before bed is a good idea. Heavy meals within an hour or two of bedtime, however, may interfere with sleep.

Step 7: Cut the Caffeine (and Nix the Nicotine, while you're at it)

Your child should avoid caffeine altogether, but definitely for at least the three to four hours before bed. Caffeine can be found in many types of soda, coffee, iced tea, and chocolate. A complete discussion of caffeine and its effects on your child, as well as a chart of how much caffeine is found in many common foods and beverages, can be found in chapter 5. Don't forget that nicotine is a stimulant, and in addition to all the other bad things that smoking can do to your teenager, it can also interfere with her sleep.

Step 8: Cut the Cord

We admit, this advice is not for everyone. We are very sensitive to the fact that parents may choose to have their children sleep with them instead of by themselves, and that in many cultures this practice is perfectly acceptable. However, if you do want your child to sleep independently (and there are some very good reasons why this might be a better choice for you and your child), you need to make sure he is able to fall asleep on his own. All children naturally awaken during the night. However, whatever your child needs to fall asleep at bedtime is what he'll need to fall back to sleep during the night. So if you are lying down with your child at bedtime, he'll need you next to him again when he wakes up during the night. (See chapter 9 for more advice on how to help your child fall asleep and stay asleep on his own.)

Step 9: See the Light

Have your child spend time outside every day, especially in the morning, as exposure to sunlight, or bright light, helps to keep the body's internal clock on track. This is especially important for night owls and adolescents who tend to let their internal clock shift later.

Step 10: Know Your Naps

Naps should be geared to your child's age and developmental needs. However, very long naps or too many naps should be avoided, as too much daytime sleep can result in your child sleeping less at night.

For a teenager who occasionally does not get enough sleep at night, a thirty- to forty-five-minute nap in the early afternoon can be beneficial. However, this strategy is *not* a long-term substitute for getting enough sleep at night. Don't let the nap be too long or too late in the afternoon, or your adolescent will have difficulty falling asleep at bedtime.

What Else Can I Do?

These suggestions are pretty much one-size-fits-all; in other words, they apply equally well to nearly all kids. But what about finding solutions that fit your child's special sleep personality (see chapter 2)? Just as every child and teenager has their own very unique set of temperamental characteristics, likes and dislikes, strengths and not-so-strong-points, the same goes for sleep patterns. And some of these sleep patterns seem to have features in common that make for distinct sleep personality types, which call for some special handling. You might just recognize your child in one of the descriptions below.

The Princess (Prince) and the Pea

Sleep Personality Profile: These young ladies (or gentlemen) seem extraordinarily sensitive to just about any aspect of the sleeping environment you can name, including the degree of light, noise, and temperature in the room; the firmness of their mattress; the number of pillows they use; the color of their pajamas; and the required number of stories at bedtime. Sleep problems, when they arise, are most likely to be related to changes in the sleeping environment; for example, these kids may have particular problems sleeping away from home, or when there are extremes in temperature, or even for a week or two after the daylight savings time switch.

Sleep Strategies: Make sure your little princess has her own pillow, favorite pj's, normal bedtime snack, and so forth whenever you travel. As much as possible, anticipate potential sleep environment changes (like daylight savings time). Environmental controls such as air conditioners, white noise machines, and eyeshades or room-darkening shades may be particularly helpful to these children. A regular bedtime routine is also very important, but here's a word of caution: it's easy to fall into the ever-expanding, never-ending bedtime-rituals trap with these kids, because they seem so dependent on them to fall asleep, so be sure to set limits ahead of time.

The Energizer Bunny

Sleep Personality Profile: These are the kids who appear to be able to keep going and going and going, long past the point at which everyone else around them has dropped. Naps are not part of their vocabulary. And when they finally do run out of steam, they are also likely to go from sixty miles an hour to fast asleep in a matter of minutes. Often they are not only the first ones up in the morning, but they are also disgustingly cheerful and ready to face the day, no matter what time they've gone to bed the night before. Some of these kids may truly need *somewhat* less sleep (see chapter 4) than the rest of us mortals, or they may be a little better able to handle not getting quite enough sleep. But ironically, for some kids, their seemingly extraordinary energy level may actually be an indication that they are "overtired" and in fact, need *more* sleep.

Sleep Strategies: The key here is not to assume your little perpetual motion machine was "just born that way" and is indeed getting enough sleep. Look for clues like the child's level of energy ("hyperactive" vs. "active"), irritability, and moodiness that might suggest a lack of sleep. Kids who need more sleep are also likely to become *most active* at those times when you would expect them to be *most tired* (i.e., bedtime) and are also likely to nod off as soon as they are not able to run around (for example, on long car rides).

Assuming that lack of sleep is not an issue for your active child, the challenge becomes mustering up enough energy yourself to keep up with him. Bedtime may need to be adjusted a bit to coincide with your child's natural "crash" time. Don't be tempted to use electronic means (TV) to try to get him to fall asleep. Tips for dealing with an early riser are found in chapter 7.

The Rock Star

Sleep Personality Profile: These adolescents have most likely been "night owls" from day one. Once puberty hits, however, their lifestyle on weekends increasingly begins to resemble that of your average heavy metal band—up all night, sleep all day. These teens tend to crash hard and crash wherever they happen to be, generally fully clothed, on the couch, with the TV blaring. They may even gradually gravitate toward setting up a permanent bedroom shop in the basement, where the cavelike atmosphere is less likely to interfere with sleeping till noon. In extreme cases, mealtimes on weekends become random events and family interactions during daylight hours are pretty minimal (unless you count grunts as conversation).

Sleep Strategies: The key here is to see the handwriting on the wall in cases where this behavior is starting to interfere with other things in life, such as going to school, doing homework, and being a semi-participating member of a family. Chapter 18 explores some of the mysterious world of adolescent sleep and should help you start to figure out what's normal and what's not. The bottom line is, it's your job as a parent to monitor your teenager's sleep habits (at least until she goes away to college and can take afternoon classes).

The Grouch

Sleep Personality Profile: These children seem to be particularly sensitive to the effects of not getting as much sleep as they need. They are easy to pick out of the crowd on the morning after a sleepover party, because they're so cranky. They have a terrible time getting dressed, organized, and out the door on days when they haven't slept well. Usually upbeat and smiling, they become short-tempered, grouchy, and sullen when not well rested, but they just as quickly revert to their cheerful selves after a good night's sleep.

Sleep Strategies: If this sounds like your child, what you as a parent can do is to make sure your child gets as much sleep as she needs. This is fairly simple when kids are younger, but obviously more of a challenge as other priorities begin to surface in later childhood and adolescence. See chapters 5 and 7 for tips on identifying potential sleep thieves and on dealing with situations like sleepovers and too many activities.

Garfield Jr.

Sleep Personality Profile: Like the legendary feline, some kids truly love to sleep and are really good at it. They are also very good at managing to get sleep when they need it (whenever the son of one of the authors was out at a restaurant with his negligent parents when bedtime arrived, would carefully put two dining chairs together, wad up his jacket for a pillow, and go to sleep—a true sleep prodigy, even as a toddler). These are the kids who announce in the middle of a TV show that they are tired and take themselves off to bed. And once asleep, they usually continue to sleep through all manner of noise, chaos, and interruptions (this same young man would typically fall asleep with the overhead light in his bedroom blazing with approximately operating-room intensity).

Sleep Strategies: If you are fortunate enough to be the parent of one of these sleep geniuses, you don't need to do a whole lot except keep out of their way and thank your lucky stars. And don't feel too smug, as your next child will most likely be the complete opposite (you don't get more than one of these to a family).

7

"What Do I Do?":
The Top Parenting Sleep Challenges

Every parent has faced some challenges when it comes to the subject of sleep. It could be dealing with sleepovers, handling a child who seems to open up to talk only when it's way past bedtime, or getting a sleepy teen out of bed in the morning for school. Compiled here are the top sleep dilemmas that parents face and a discussion of ways to manage them. Just as with many parenting issues, there are no perfect solutions for many of these dilemmas, but suggestions are provided to help you negotiate such issues.

Setting Priorities

The most common theme in terms of sleep challenges is setting priorities—that is, balancing the need for sleep versus the demands of life. There is no question that it is difficult to maintain a balance between the importance of sleep and other priorities in life. Do you sacrifice sleep to go to the soccer tournament? Do you have your son finish his homework even though it's already past 10:00 at night? It may not have been his fault; the assignment just took longer than expected. Do you let your daughter stay up late to finish reading a book just because it's really good?

How do you strike a balance? We all know that good nutrition, exercise, and sleep are important for good health, but we constantly make choices about how important they are at any given point in time depending on what else takes precedence. Of course, good nutrition goes out the window at times like birthday parties and Halloween. Sleep can also go out the window on New Year's Eve, for a night out to the circus, for a family wedding, and for sleepovers. But on a daily basis, where do you draw the line, and what are the priorities? How do you live a healthy life (with a good dose of sleep) that is also sane and realistic? And, finally, how do you accomplish this within the context of childhood development issues, such as the need for increasing independence as your child becomes a teenager? As you consider this balance, note that at first you need to make these decisions for your child, but as your child gets older, you have to teach them how to do it for themselves.

Sleepovers

Jessica is mother to two girls, ages ten and eight. Both daughters get invited to lots of sleepovers. It's fun for the girls, but they are usually extremely tired the next day and "off" sometimes into the next week. It's a major complaint among the parents in her daughters' circles of friends.

Sleepovers are fun, but they are also notorious for leading to next-day exhaustion. They probably should be called "stay-awake-overs" instead. However, sleepovers are often an important part of a child's social life.

Below are different ways that sleepovers can be handled so that fun can be had without too high a price being paid in terms of exhaustion. As one mother put it, "Sleepovers can be great for everyone or a disaster for everyone." Plan ahead so that the fun aspect wins out.

- **Set a lights-out time.** Let the kids know right from the beginning what time lights need to go out and the "no talking" rule takes over. Lights out can be one hour past your child's usual bedtime or some other predetermined time. The term "usual bedtime" may need to be negotiated. Is it the usual bedtime of your child or the usual bedtime of the other child?
- **Play the part of sleep police.** Let the kids know there will be no exceptions or changes to the lights-out rule. So if they arrive at 7:00 PM and know that the lights-out time is 11:00 PM they'd better squeeze in all the fun they can in that time frame. As one mother said, "I usually have to police the area a bit after lights-out, just for those who haven't taken my 'no talking' admonition seriously . . . but generally I've had no problem."

- **Set consequences.** Let the kids know there are consequences to continuing to talk after the "no talking" rule begins. For example, maybe the next sleepover won't happen or they won't get a special breakfast treat.
- **Limit the frequency of sleepovers.** You know your child best, so you know what he can handle. Some children can handle one sleepover night each weekend, whereas others can handle sleepovers only on special occasions. Limit sleepovers to what works best for your child and for your family. Talk with your child about the impact of sleepovers and decide together which ones are important and whether he can "afford" to go.
- **Make sleepovers special events.** Rather than sleepovers being a regular occasion, save them for special events when your child gets to stay up really late (like New Year's Eve) and everyone just pays the consequences of sleep deprivation the next day (parents and kids).
- **Have an "almost-sleepover."** Have your child stay at a friend's house just until bedtime and then come home. This way your child can have the fun of hanging out all night with his friend(s) but still get a good night's sleep. For a middle-school or high-school student, this may be coming home as late as midnight or 1:00 AM. Invite your child's friend(s) over, too, for an "almost sleepover."
- **Schedule naptime the next day.** On days after a sleepover, schedule a nap for your child. This will allow your child to have sleepovers but still get the sleep he needs.
- **Negotiate common rules among parents.** If your child has a group of friends who often have sleepovers at each other's houses, discuss the issue with the other parents and come up with some common rules, including how often sleepovers occur and a standard lights-out time across all the families.

Reading in Bed

Many nights, Hannah's parents find her reading under the covers with a flashlight. When they go to check on her, they hear some fast rustling as she tries to quickly hide the flashlight and the book. Her parents hate telling her to stop reading, but they also want her to get the sleep she needs.

"My biggest challenge right now is convincing Joe to go to bed at a decent hour. He's fifteen, and he wants to stay up until 11:00 PM or midnight every school night, and then (of course) has to get up by 6:00 AM to make the bus at 6:45. He's usually just reading at the point that I finally say, "Okay, that's it—lights out!" and I hate to have to tell him to stop reading. He just says he doesn't feel tired at 9:00 or 10:00 PM."

Obviously, reading is very important and all parents want to support literacy in their child. What's a parent to do, then, when it's time for lights-out but your child wants to read? In most cases, a compromise is in order. Move your child's bedtime routine earlier by about a half-hour and let your child stay up in bed reading until it's lights-out time. Another way is to rearrange your bedtime routine so that plenty of reading time is included. For example, move taking a nighttime shower to right before or after dinner or in the morning so there is more time to read in the evening. You can also give your child an extra fifteen to thirty minutes of reading time for a slightly later lights-out time. Again, it's all about balancing priorities.

Now She Wants to Talk!

The only quiet time in the Lewis household is at bedtime, when all the kids are snugly tucked into bed. For Michelle, this is the only time that she has one-on-one time with her mother. The rest of the day is hectic, with her and her two siblings always on the go to different activities and vying for their parents' attention. The family tries to eat dinner together every night, but it's not the time for a heart-to-heart discussion. So, often her parents find that it's not until 9:00 at night when Michelle starts telling them what is really going on with her.

The problem that Tricia has with her son Christopher, who is seven, is that he always waits until bedtime to tell her what happened to him at school that day. She certainly wants to hear about his day, but not at 9:30 at night, when he should be asleep.

There are many reasons why children and teenagers wait until bedtime to finally tell their parents about their day. It may be the only quiet moment in a hectic household. It may be a stalling tactic, to keep going to sleep at bay. It may be that your child has finally processed what has happened and is just now ready to talk about it.

Try building into your child's bedtime at least five to ten minutes of time to connect. Rather than rushing through the bedtime routine and heading out the door right away, stay put and talk about what is going on. Many times it will be a simple conversation about what happened that day and what's going to happen tomorrow. But by laying the foundation and setting aside the time, you will find that your child will likely open up when he needs to. And this way, you won't be frustrated when your child wants to talk, as it's already built into the schedule.

If you have more than one child, it may seem difficult to find the time, but it will be worth it. During one's "talking time," the other child can be reading or looking at books in bed. Spend time with your younger one first, so that her bedtime doesn't get delayed, giving your older one a slightly later bedtime.

Night Owls

Terry, age nine, is a total night owl. No matter what time her parents put her to bed and turn out the lights, she is still awake at 11:00 PM. And, of course, she is tired the next day.

There really are children who are night owls and others who are morning larks. The night owls are energized in the evening, have a hard time falling asleep early, and can sleep much later in the morning than others their age. The larks are ready to head for bed by 8:00 or 9:00 and happy to see the day first thing in the morning. To help determine if your child is an owl or a lark, see chapter 15.

The most important thing to help night owls is not to let them drift too much on weekends and on vacations. On weekends, it's best to let them stay up later on only one of the nights. And even then, try to not let them stay up more than an hour past their usual bedtime. The other important thing is to wake them up in the morning, again not letting them sleep much later than they usually do on weekdays. Our internal clocks are governed mostly by what time we wake up in the morning, so letting your night owl sleep in will keep his internal clock shifted later and make it difficult for him to fall asleep at a reasonable hour that night.

Note that the internal clocks of some night owls may shift so much that they develop delayed sleep phase syndrome. See chapter 15 on identifying and treating this sleep disorder.

Waking Up Too Early

Jennifer is the mother of two preschoolers, ages four and five. No matter what time the children go to bed, they are up before dawn, usually between 5:30 and 6:00. They have not gotten enough sleep and are crabby by 8:00. Their mother has tried telling them to go back to sleep, she has tried laying down with them, and in her words, "I've even considered a sledge hammer." For about a week, she got them to agree to stay by themselves and not wake her up, but it didn't last.

There are two groups of children who wake up too early in the morning. The first group is those who have gotten enough sleep and are wide-awake, ready to start the day. Most of these children are early birds. By the age of five or six, most early birds are independent enough to be up alone and not wake up everyone else in the family. Be clear about what your child is allowed to do, though, while everyone else is still sleeping (for example, giving the dog a haircut is presumably not on the list of acceptable activities). Does he need to stay in his room, where he may play with his toys? Can he lie in bed and read? Some families put out breakfast for their child (a bowl of cereal and a juice box) in the family room, where their child can watch television until everyone else is up. You can also set an alarm to let your child know when he is allowed to come into your room.

The other group is those who wake up early but have not gotten enough sleep. For some children, there is something that is waking them up, such as being too cold, a local garbage truck that makes its rounds at 5:00 AM, or morning light streaming in the bedroom window. Try to solve these problems first—turn up the heat, put a white noise machine in your child's room, and add room-darkening shades. For others, it's actually the final night waking but your child has slept enough by that point that it makes it hard to fall back to sleep. Check out chapter 9 on what causes night wakings and how to deal with them.

Sleeping with Parents

Gregory is seven years old and sleeps in his parents' room every night. He prefers to sleep in bed with them, but in the past six months they have gotten him to sleep on a sleeping bag on their bedroom floor. In the past, he has slept in his own room. His parents aren't sure whether to let him keep sleeping in their room.

Children who sleep with their parents are quite common, especially worldwide. In about two-thirds of countries the majority of children sleep with their parents, at least until the age of three or four. However, in the United States, and other industrialized countries, children are much more likely to sleep in their own room, separate from their parents.

Whether you have your child sleep with you—either in your bed or in your room—is a family decision that you need to make. The most important consideration is to first figure out the reason that your child sleeps with you. If it is because it's the only sleeping space that you have, then that's the way it is. If your child is sleeping with you because of personal and family values that you believe children should share a sleeping space with their parents, then again it is appropriate and there is no reason to make a change. However, do note that in our culture, older children (older than about age three or four) are expected to sleep independently, and children may start to feel different from their friends and classmates if they continue to share a bed or a room with their parents. Also, as children get above the age of about six, they will start to want some privacy and their own space.

There are other reasons that children sleep with their parents that may indicate that a change is appropriate.

- **Behavioral habit.** Some children, even as old as ten or twelve years, have a habit of requiring a parent to be present to help them fall asleep at bedtime or back to sleep during the night. Chapter 9 gives much more information on this issue, but basically children all learn to fall asleep in some particular way, and that habit becomes ingrained. These habits are called *sleep associations*. The sleep association will need to be present at bedtime and during the night after a normal nighttime arousal. So your child's sleep association may literally be you. If your child has been sleeping with you for a long time, and if either of you want to make a change, take it slowly. A gradual change over a few weeks isn't going to matter. Start by working on just bedtime and having your child fall asleep independently. Or start by moving both of you into your child's room, so he gets used to sleeping in his own bed all night. Once your child is comfortable sleeping in his own room, you can then begin easing yourself out—such as staying for a few minutes at bedtime and during the night but not sleeping there the entire night. By the time your child is school-aged, he may be quite motivated to make this change so he can start thinking about sleepovers at his friends' and feel like a "big kid." Even so, take it slow so that he doesn't feel like a failure if all doesn't go totally smoothly while making the change.

- **Anxiety.** Many school-aged children who have an underlying anxiety issue are too anxious to be alone and want a parent with them at bedtime and throughout the night. Children who co-sleep because of anxiety are usually anxious at other times of the day, too. For example, they may be nervous about being alone in parts of the house without someone else there. They may refuse to go upstairs alone. They may get anxious about going to places such as school, a friend's house, or sports practice without a parent or someone else they are comfortable with. Children who are anxious usually worry more than other children their age. If your child is sleeping with you because of anxiety, the best thing to do is to seek help about anxiety issues first. Your child needs to develop coping skills to deal with the anxiety before any changes surrounding sleep can be made. (For more information on sleep and anxiety, see chapter 19.)

Bearding the Lion in the Bedroom: "We Can't Get Her Up in the Morning"

"High school starts around 7:30 where we live, and getting up at 6:00 or 6:30 is pure torture for my daughter—and by extension for both of us. She literally has two alarm clocks that she manages to sleep through, forcing us to repeatedly come in and wake her up ourselves. Every morning, John and I argue about whose turn it is to venture into the lion's cage—more

often than not, a simple wake-up call is met with the verbal equivalent of a mauling. It really doesn't matter how early she goes to bed, the morning is just never her best time."

Getting a sleepy child or teenager up in the morning can be a daunting task, and one that is all too familiar to many families. Difficulty getting up in the morning is almost always a result of not getting enough sleep. It can also be part of being a night owl, who doesn't feel his best until the evening. As one night owl put it, "You mean there are two seven o'clocks in a day?" Below are some tips for getting your anti-morning child up and out of bed:

- **Go to bed earlier.** Yes, this is an obvious answer. But if you can get your child to go to bed earlier, even if it's only every other night, it's going to make a world of difference.
- **Open the shades.** Light is what alerts us in the morning. Physiologically, light suppresses melatonin, the naturally produced hormone that makes us feel sleepy. Exposure to light will decrease the level of this sleep-inducing hormone and help your child wake up in the morning. So open the shades or turn on a bedroom light. It's even better if you can open the shades about thirty minutes before your child needs to wake up.
- **Skip the snooze button.** What teens (and adults) often do is set their alarm clock much earlier than needed so that they can keep hitting the snooze button. This is a misguided attempt to steal a few extra minutes of sleep. Instead, what it basically does is ruin the last part of your night's sleep. So stop having your teen set his alarm clock early. Instead, set it for the time that he really does have to get up in the morning, or at the most so that he only has time to hit the snooze button once.
- **Put the alarm clock across the room.** If your child at least hears the alarm clock and turns it off himself, put it across the room. Having to get up and cross the room to turn it off is a surefire way to get him out of bed. Also, set the alarm clock to the most annoying sound possible, rather than to a classical musical station that will simply lull him back to sleep.

She Doesn't Get Enough Sleep

Alexa is fifteen years old, and she clearly doesn't get enough sleep. According to her mother, "She is lucky to get seven to eight hours on weekdays. She's tired and cranky, especially by the end of the week. On weekends, she'll often sleep until 11:00 or 12:00, which cuts into the day, but she really needs it to catch up from the week."

Not getting enough sleep is standard for most adolescents today. The average teenager gets between seven and seven and a half hours of sleep, when they actually need nine to nine and a half hours. Chapter 18 discusses this national epidemic of sleepy teenagers, the reasons for it, and ways that families can help their teens get enough sleep.

If your child is not a teenager yet, there are still some things that you can do to ensure that she is getting the sleep that she needs. Chapter 6 provides the ten steps to a good night's sleep. In addition, you need to help restructure your child's day to set bedtime much earlier so that she gets the sleep she needs.

Sleep: It's Not Just for Kids

Children and adolescents are not the only ones who have sleep problems. Parents experience them too. In fact, 70 million Americans struggle with sleep problems. There are a number of common adult sleep problems, and we cover the four most common ones here—insomnia, sleep apnea, restless legs syndrome, and periodic limb movement disorder. But, most importantly, maintaining good sleep habits can make a world of difference.

Good Sleep Habits

Just like it's important for your child to have good sleep habits, you should too.

- **Put sleep at the top of (or at least on) your "to do" list.** Just as sleep is important for children and adolescents, sleep is essential for adults too. Structure your day so that you can get the sleep that you need. You'll be surprised at how much better you feel, and how much more efficient you are, if you get enough sleep. Rather than getting less done, you will actually get more done in a day. You will also be a good sleep role model for your children.

- **Stay regular.** Go to bed at the same time every night, and wake up at the same time every morning. This can be difficult to do, but it will help set your internal clock and make it easier for you to fall asleep and stay asleep.
- **Stick to a routine.** As is true for your child, a bedtime routine is a way to help your body know that it is time to sleep. Include something relaxing as part of your bedtime routine, such as taking a bath, reading a book, or listening to soothing music.
- **Avoid naps if you have trouble sleeping.** If you are having problems sleeping, avoid taking a daytime nap. Taking a nap can interfere with falling asleep at bedtime and staying asleep.
- **Skip the caffeine late in the day.** Avoid caffeine, at least for the three to four hours before you go to bed. For some people it's best to even avoid it after lunch. A listing of caffeinated products and how much caffeine they contain is provided in chapter 5.
- **Don't smoke, don't drink.** Like all stimulants, the nicotine found in cigarettes (cigars, pipe and chewing tobacco, etc.) disrupts sleep, making it difficult to fall asleep and stay asleep (it's also not good for you!). Alcohol also disrupts sleep. Although its sedating effect may make it easier for you to fall asleep at night, a nightcap can leads to disrupted sleep later on, as the alcohol effects wear off toward the early morning hours. If you can't give up these bad habits altogether, at least try not to smoke after dinner and avoid alcohol later in the evening.
- **Feel the burn.** Exercise can help you get a better night's sleep. However, avoid exercising too close to bedtime. It's better to exercise at least several hours before it's time to head to bed.
- **Eat light.** A light snack before bed can avoid bedtime and middle-of-the-night hunger. On the other hand, avoid eating a heavy meal close to bedtime.
- **Make your bedroom "sleep-friendly."** Just as you've done for your child, set up your bedroom so that it is conducive to sleep. To ensure a good night's sleep, make it cool, dark, and quiet. Get a mattress and pillow that are comfortable. If street noise awakens you, run a white noise maker or a fan to drown out the sounds.

Also get the television out of your bedroom. Move your desk to another space so that you are not staring at your pile of bills as you climb into bed. Move the computer out so that you are not tempted to check your e-mail one last time.

Insomnia

"Now I Can't Sleep!"

After several years of struggling to get her toddler to sleep through the night, Janine ended up with major sleep problems herself. She had always been the "best sleeper in the world, in love with sleep, able to sleep anywhere, anytime." But for whatever reason, she now finds it impossible to sleep. Janine has been struggling with this issue for the past four years.

Insomnia is one of the most common sleep problems experienced by adults. Insomnia can involve difficulty falling asleep, waking during the night, or waking too early in the morning. Insomnia also usually involves feeling tired the next day. There are many causes of insomnia. Sometimes insomnia is a symptom of something else. For example, insomnia can be the result of depression, anxiety, or another sleep disorder such as sleep apnea or restless legs syndrome. It can be caused by pain, a medical condition, or a medication.

Most of the time, though, the insomnia itself is the problem. The insomnia usually starts as a result of some life event, whether it's the birth of a child, an illness, or a change in job. It is then perpetuated by negative thoughts about sleep and poor sleep habits that develop to counteract the sleeplessness, such as spending too much time in bed, napping during the day, and sleeping in on days off.

There are many resources available to adults about how to deal with insomnia. Appendix B provides a list of books on adult sleep that can be helpful, as well as a list of other resources. Your doctor or local sleep center can also be very helpful.

SEVEN RULES FOR BEATING INSOMNIA

1. **Choose a set wake-up time.** Wake up at exactly the same time every day, no matter how much sleep you got the night before.

2. **Choose a bedtime.** Pick a bedtime that enables you to get the sleep you need. However, spending too much time in bed will lead to more interrupted sleep, so the best bedtime is one that allows you to get the sleep that you need but doesn't let you be in bed too long. You want to spend only the amount of time in bed that you actually need for sleep.

3. **Go to bed when you are sleepy, but not before your chosen bedtime.** Don't go to bed until you are sleepy. If you are still not sleepy at your chosen bedtime, wait until you are sleepy. This will help you to fall asleep quickly.

4. **Get out of bed when you can't sleep.** If you are lying in bed and can't sleep, get out of bed and do something relaxing. It's best to leave your bedroom. Read a book or do something else relaxing; then go back to bed when you feel sleepy. Again, if you do not fall asleep quickly, get up. Keep repeating this cycle until you fall asleep. You need to get out of bed when you can't sleep at bedtime and in the middle of the night (that's the hard part!).

5. **Don't worry or plan in bed.** When lying in bed at night, don't worry or plan for the next day. Set aside another time of the day to do these things. If you start thinking and worrying when you get in bed, get up. Don't head back to bed until you feel your thoughts won't interfere with falling asleep. Thinking in bed is a habit, and one that you can break.

6. **Use your bed for sleep only.** Don't do anything but sleep in your bed. That is, don't do other activities, such as eat, watch television, or pay bills, in your bed (romance is allowed, of course).

7. **Avoid naps.** If you have insomnia, taking a nap will make it difficult to fall asleep at bedtime. So, no naps.

Sleep Apnea

Snoring and sleep apnea are common in adults, primarily in overweight middle-age men and in postmenopausal women. However, anyone can develop sleep apnea, which involves repetitive episodes of upper airway obstruction. This means that you stop breathing repeatedly throughout the night. Sleep apnea can be serious, as it results in significant sleepiness the next day and can have long-term health implications.

SYMPTOMS OF SLEEP APNEA

- Snoring

- Breathing pauses

- Coughing and choking during sleep

- Daytime sleepiness

- Morning headache

- Dry mouth

- Restless sleep

- Insomnia

There are a number of treatment options available for sleep apnea in adults. The most appropriate treatment for you will depend on the severity of your sleep apnea, what factors may be contributing to your sleep apnea, and what will work best for you. A common treatment is *nasal CPAP* (continuous positive airway pressure). This involves wearing a mask over the nose while you sleep. Air pressure from a compressor is forced down the nose, keeping the airway open. Other treatments include surgery, dental appliances, weight loss, and medications. If you think that you or someone you know has sleep apnea, you should definitely talk with your doctor.

Restless Legs Syndrome and Periodic Limb Movement Disorder

Restless legs syndrome (RLS) is a creepy-crawly feeling in the legs that usually occurs when lying down to go to sleep. It can also occur at other times of inactivity, such as while riding in a car or watching a movie. There is usually an uncontrollable urge to move the legs to alleviate the uncomfortable feeling. As you can imagine, this results in difficulty falling asleep. RLS is relatively common, affecting between 5 and 15 percent of adults. RLS is also more common during pregnancy. About 80 percent of adults with RLS also have periodic limb movement disorder (PLMD).

Periodic limb movement disorder (PLMD) is a sleep disorder in which a person's limbs, usually the legs, repeatedly jerk or kick during sleep. You may or may not be aware of these movements. Rather, you may get complaints from a bed partner that you are an extremely restless sleeper, and you may experience daytime sleepiness the next day although you seemingly got enough sleep the prior night. Many people with PLMS are unaware of their problem.

A sleep specialist typically diagnoses RLS and PLMS. There are treatments available for this disorder, primarily medication-based. Both caffeine and alcohol can exacerbate these two conditions, so be sure to avoid them. An iron deficiency can also be the cause of these two sleep disorders, so your doctor may check for anemia.

PART THREE: SLEEP PROBLEMS AND SOLUTIONS

8

"I'm Not Going To Bed": Bedtime Problems

"Every night around 8:00, while Stefan is quietly playing, I begin to dread the ordeal of bedtime. The next thing I know it is 9:30 and Stefan is overtired. Now it becomes impossible to get him to bed without a fight. By the time he is finally asleep, it is 10:30 and I am tense and exhausted. This is not the life I envisioned."

Getting a child to go to bed is the most common sleep problem that parents face. Some children resist going to bed by stalling and finding excuses, while others go to bed initially but then do not stay there. Almost half of all preschoolers and school-aged children stall at bedtime, with many refusing to go to bed altogether. So if your child does this, realize that you are not alone. Bedtime can be one of the most frustrating parts of a parent's day.

What Bedtime Problems May Look Like

There are many different ways that children can give their parents a hard time at bedtime. Below are just a few (maybe one of these scenarios will seem a lot like your house!):

- **Stalling at bedtime.** Your child may be the master (or mistress) at stalling at bedtime, attempting to delay bedtime by asking to watch "just one more television show" or delay lights-out with "just one more story" or "five more minutes, *please!*"

- **Refusing to go to bed.** Your child may literally refuse to get ready for bed or go to bed. He may refuse to change into his pajamas, brush his teeth, or get into his bed, let alone stay there. He may follow you back to the living room, refusing to stay in his room.
- **Resisting going to bed.** Rather than outright refusing, your child may fight you every step of the way or need you to stay with him at bedtime.
- **"Curtain calls."** Your child may be fine about going to bed, but then start incessant requests after you have already left the room—asking for another drink, another hug and kiss, to have her covers straightened, or whatever other request she can think of.
- **Refusing to sleep in her own room.** Another common problem is that your child sleeps someplace other than her own room or own bed. For example, your child may be able to fall asleep only while watching television in the living room or when she is in your bed. She may frequently sneak into a sibling's room and sleep there.
- **Taking a long time to fall asleep.** A final bedtime issue is taking a long time to fall asleep once the lights are turned out. About 20 percent of children take more than twenty minutes to fall asleep. Check out chapter 11 on insomnia if this describes your child.

HE HAS NO PROBLEM WHEN . . .

Some children won't go to bed for anyone, but there are many children who will go to sleep quickly for others, such as for a babysitter, grandmother, or for one parent but not the other. This is often an indication that the parent for whom your child is difficult needs to do a better job of setting limits, having clear bedtime rules and providing clear consequences.

Your child may also not have problems falling asleep at bedtime in places that are not his bedroom, such as on the couch watching television. This is often an indication that your child doesn't literally have problems falling asleep at night, but rather that something else is going on.

How Common Is It?

Although bedtime problems can occur at any age, they are most common in children who are between three and six years old. A recent National Sleep Foundation poll found that 52 percent of preschoolers and 42 percent of school-aged children stall at bedtime. In addition, one out of three preschoolers and 14 percent of school-aged children resist going to bed. Bedtime resistance in adolescents is an altogether different animal (in teenagers, isn't everything?) and is covered in chapter 18.

Causes

There are many reasons that children have problems at bedtime. Some potential reasons include:

- **Parenting style.** A common cause of noncompliance at bedtime is parenting style. Parents who are more permissive or have problems setting limits and disciplining their child are more likely to have a child who has bedtime issues.

  Andrea has two daughters—Sarah, who is three and a half, and Jenna, who is four and a half. They have little structure to their day and are usually in their shared bedroom by 10:00 PM. They watch television and eventually fall asleep anytime between 11:00 PM and 2:00 AM. Both girls are cranky and irritable the next day.

- **Conflicting parenting discipline styles.** When parents have different styles, especially when parents frequently disagree about how to handle behavior problems, behavioral issues may flourish. In this situation, one parent is often strict, while the other is more lenient, basically a "good cop/bad cop" scenario. Children often sense (and sometimes exploit) these differences, which leads to more noncompliant behavior and often lots of family disagreements.
- **Age.** As simplistic as it sounds, age can be a factor. Younger children, especially preschoolers, are more likely to assert their independence and refuse to comply with their parents' requests. As

children get older, they typically require less reminding and prodding and are more compliant about going to bed.

- **Temperament.** Your child may simply be a kid who has a hard time transitioning from a busy, active day to slowing down enough to fall asleep. This can contribute to bedtime problems.
- **Sleep environment.** Sometimes your child's sleep environment may contribute to bedtime problems. For example, brothers and sisters sharing a room can cause problems. Siblings have a tendency to keep each other up at bedtime. It also may be more difficult for parents to set limits when lenient grandparents are living in the house or nearby.
- **Internal clocks.** If your child's bedtime is too early, he may not be sleepy enough to head to bed and fall asleep at bedtime. On the other hand, some children are so overtired by the time bedtime finally arrives that they are too wound up to settle down and go to sleep. So make sure you are attentive to your child's natural sleep onset time (part of his "sleep personality"), which may be later or earlier than what time you would like him to go to bed.
- **Family tension.** Bedtime problems often result in significant family tension, including arguments between you and your child, and arguments between parents. This tension, however, may lead to your child becoming anxious and agitated, making falling asleep even more difficult.

Danny has always given his parents a hard time about going to bed. Sometimes things get so bad that his parents yell at him and threaten to take away his favorite toys if he doesn't get to bed right away. This often backfires. Danny gets so distressed about possibly losing his toys that he becomes distraught, making falling asleep impossible.

What Else Could It Be?

There are other factors that may also make it difficult for your child at bedtime. Some of these include:

- **Poor sleep schedule.** As your child gets older, naps, including napping too late in the afternoon, may result in your child's not being able to fall asleep until much later in the evening. In addition, not having a regular sleep schedule, such as having varying bedtimes and wake times, can contribute to difficulties falling asleep. Similarly, it will be much more difficult to fall asleep on Sunday evenings if your child or teenager goes to bed much later on weekend nights and sleeps in on Saturday and Sunday mornings.
- **More general behavior problems.** Your child may be oppositional in general, making noncompliance at bedtime more likely. This is really a more general behavior management problem rather than a bedtime problem per se.
- **Anxiety.** Some children who have a difficult time at bedtime are actually anxious. They are too scared, too worried, or too anxious to go to bed and be alone. Typically, if a parent remains with an anxious child at bedtime, the resistance disappears and the child falls asleep relatively quickly. If you think your child is having problems with anxiety, either during the day or at night, definitely talk with a professional about it.
- **It's a phase.** Some children go through a temporary period of having problems at bedtime. These short-term sleep problems may be the result of sleeping in a new environment or one that is not conducive to sleep, such as being too hot or too noisy. It may also relate to a recent stressful event, a recent disruption in the child's sleep schedule (such as from a trip or jet lag), or a recent illness. Sticking to the same bedtime and bedtime routine will typically solve this type of problem rather quickly.
- **Delayed sleep phase syndrome.** Some children have a tendency to be night owls, but in some cases they actually have delayed sleep phase syndrome, in which their entire internal clock is shifted much later (see chapter 15 for more information). These children usually fall asleep at about the same time every night, and if bedtime gets moved close to this time, there are few problems.
- **Restless legs syndrome.** Restless legs syndrome can lead to bedtime problems. Restless legs syndrome is a neurological disorder that

causes a child (or an adult) to have uncomfortable feelings in the legs that makes it hard to lie still and to fall asleep. (For more information about restless legs syndrome, see chapter 14.)

- **Medication effects.** There are many medications that can disrupt sleep, especially stimulant medications that are given for ADHD (although some children actually do better with a late afternoon or evening dose). If your child is taking any medications, talk with his or her doctor about its impact on sleep.

IMPACT ON THE WHOLE FAMILY

Improving your child's sleep will have a positive effect across the board. Not only will your child feel better getting more sleep, but so will the entire family. Once your child is sleeping, the whole family will be sleeping. Also, there will be a huge decrease in stress for everyone.

What You Can Do to Help Your Child Go to Bed

First of all, it is important to realize that you cannot "make" your child go to sleep, but you can help your child improve his bedtime behavior and help him to fall asleep more easily and quickly. As with many other skills your child needs to learn, this will take time.

- **Maintain good sleep habits.** The first place to start is to make sure that your child has good sleep habits (see chapter 6). Be sure your child avoids caffeine and gets regular exercise. And remove that television from his bedroom!
- **Establish clear bedtime rules.** Be very clear about what is involved in getting ready for bed, such as changing into pajamas and brushing teeth. Also, let your child know what are appropriate and inappropriate bedtime behaviors. Staying in bed is appropriate, whereas calling out for another drink is not appropriate.
- **Stick to firm bedtime limits.** You must first be convinced that your child needs to change his bedtime behavior, and that setting and sticking to firm bedtime limits is in everyone's best interest, especially

your child's. Setting limits is an important part of parenting. Children do not always have a lot of self-control, so they benefit from the structure of limits that you set for them. This helps them to learn self-control. In addition, limits relieve (not cause) anxiety in children. Finally, prepare yourself for some hard work. Changing behavior is always difficult. Your child is probably happy with bedtimes the way they are and will initially have little motivation to change. You need to be consistent, persistent, and patient.

CONSISTENCY, CONSISTENCY, CONSISTENCY

Being consistent is absolutely essential to making changes. Doing the right thing consistently is great. Doing the wrong thing consistently isn't great, but not the worst. The worst is being inconsistent. Being inconsistent is like being a slot machine. The reason people keep pumping in those quarters is that you never know when you are going to hit the jackpot. Most of the time you don't, but every once in a while you win. This is the same for your child. If you say no, no, and no the first three times that your child asks, but on the fourth, fifth, or sixth time give in, your child is going to keep trying and trying. So it's much better to say no every time or yes every time as opposed to being wishy-washy.

- **Explain the new rules to your child.** Before you start a new night-time program, sit down with your child during the day and let him know what you expect. Do not make your conversation too long or involved and do not overexplain. Ignore any negative comments by your child and avoid arguing about the new rules.
- **Set a bedtime.** Once you have decided on your child's bedtime, be *consistent* about it. Establish a regular bedtime to help set your child's internal clock. Make sure your child is ready for sleep before putting him to bed. This may seem obvious, but sometimes parents set a bedtime more for their own convenience than for their child's benefit. For example, some children's biological clocks make them more likely to be "night owls." These children may have difficulty with an earlier bedtime.

- **Temporarily set bedtime later ("bedtime fading").** Putting children to bed when they are not tired increases the likelihood of bedtime struggles. Therefore, with some children it is best to start by setting bedtime at the time they usually fall asleep and then gradually moving the bedtime earlier. When you start, you will first need to determine when your child naturally falls asleep and set this as his *temporary* bedtime. If you would like your child to go to bed at 8:30, but he usually does not fall asleep until 10:30, choose 10:30 as his temporary bedtime. This will make it easier to teach your child how to fall asleep within a short time of getting into bed. Once he is falling asleep easily and quickly at his temporary bedtime, you can start moving his bedtime earlier by fifteen minutes every few days. Be patient. If you move the bedtime back too quickly, your child may not be able to fall asleep.

- **Have a bedtime routine.** Be sure to establish a consistent bedtime routine. A bedtime routine should include calm and enjoyable activities, such as a bath and bedtime stories. Avoid stimulating, high-energy activities, such as playing outside, running around, or watching exciting television shows or videos. Make a chart of your bedtime routine to help keep your child on track. Also, having the last part of the bedtime routine be a favorite activity will help motivate your child to get ready for bed.

ENJOY BEDTIME

If you have been struggling to get your child to bed, it's safe to assume that you can't imagine actually enjoying bedtime. But that can happen. Start with adding something to your child's bedtime routine that both of you enjoy. It doesn't have to be something that traditionally happens at bedtime. It can be playing a card game, doing a crossword puzzle together, or playing make-believe. One father struggled every night to get his five-year-old son to go to bed, because all his son wanted to do was to play with action figures. Once the father added five minutes of action figure play as the last thing before lights-out, bedtime completely calmed down and his son actually looked forward to getting in bed so that they could have "guy time." For years ahead, playing "guys" at bedtime will be a wonderful memory of shared time together for both of them.

- **Provide a transitional object.** A transitional object, such as a blanket, doll, or stuffed animal, can help a child settle down and go to sleep.
- **Ignore any complaints or protests.** Ignore your child's complaints or protests about bedtime, such as not being tired. Discussing or arguing about bedtime will lead to a struggle with your child, thus perpetuating bedtime problems. Firmly and calmly let your child know it is time for bed and continue with the routine. When the bedtime routine is complete, put your child to bed and leave the room. It is important that you leave the room while your child is awake, as this helps him to learn to fall asleep on his own.
- **Check in.** If your child is yelling or calling out to you but remaining in his bed, remind him one time that it's bedtime. If he continues to be upset, check on him. Wait as long or short a time as you are comfortable with. For some children, checking frequently is effective; for others, checking infrequently works best. Continue returning to check on your child as long as he is crying or upset. The visits should be *brief* (one minute) and *boring*. Don't soothe or comfort your child during these visits, and don't get into a discussion or argument. Calmly tell him it's time to go to sleep. The purpose of returning to the room is to reassure him that you are still present and to reassure yourself that he is okay.
- **Stay calm.** If your child gets out of bed or comes out of his room, firmly and calmly return him to bed. For some children, simply returning them to bed multiple times works. For others, letting him know that if he gets up again you will close the bedroom door can be effective. If your child gets out of bed, put him back in bed and close the door for a brief period (one minute to start). After the allotted time, open the door. If your child is in bed, praise him and leave the door open. If he is up, put him back in bed and close the door again but leave it closed for a longer time, increasing the time by a few minutes each time he gets up.
- **Don't lock your child in his room.** Locking the door is scary, especially for younger children, and it is only likely to make everyone more agitated. The goal is to teach your child to stay in bed, not to punish or scare him.

- **Reward your child.** Soon after your child awakens in the morning, reward him for what he did well the night before. Don't dwell on misbehavior from the previous night. Give your attention to your child's successes. Stickers, praise, and breakfast treats are good ways to reward him for even small improvements. Larger rewards can be offered for continued positive behaviors, such as three nights of going to bed without protest. Longer-term rewards should be based on the number of successes rather than on number of consecutive nights of success (e.g., three stickers per week, not three consecutive stickers, mean a trip to the playground). Also, the reward schedule should initially be set up to ensure a reasonable expectation of immediate success, which is likely to increase your child's investment in the process.
- **Be consistent and don't give up.** The first few nights are likely to be very challenging. You should start to see major improvements within the first few weeks.
- **Expect things to get worse before they get better.** Often, things will get worse for several days before you see a significant improvement. This is because your child is going to test the rules. Be sure to stick with your plan. Once you are over the hump, you'll find that it will get easier and easier. However, don't be surprised if at times your child tries to test you again.

Diana was thrilled with how well things were going with her four-year-old son, Delonte. She was much clearer about what he needed to do to get ready for bed, and everyone was calmer and enjoying the new bedtime routine. Two weeks later, though, Delonte started demanding after lights-out that he needed to go to the bathroom. Things started to escalate again until his mother included a trip to the bathroom as the last thing that happened before lights-out and started to ignore his calling. Within a few days, things were back on track.

BEST BEHAVIOR MANAGEMENT STRATEGIES

Bedtime problems are similar to any other behavioral issue and thus respond to general behavior management strategies.

• Use positives to increase your child's appropriate behaviors.

• Avoid punishment, as it is not an effective way to change your child's behavior.

• Focus on increasing good behaviors rather than decreasing bad behaviors.

• Be consistent in responding, as this is the key to behavior change.

• Do not ask questions (e.g., "Ready for bed?") when you intend to give a command (e.g., "Time for bed.").

• Set clear limits and follow through.

• Provide acceptable choices (e.g., "Do you want to go now, or in five minutes?") to give your child some control but within reasonable limits.

9

Still Not Sleeping Through the Night: Night Wakings

Linda and John arrived at the office, looking exhausted, with their seven-year-old son, Noah. After seven years, Linda and John can recall only three nights when Noah slept through the night. They had always figured that eventually he would grow out of it. At this point, they feel as if they have given in, letting Noah come into their bed when he wakes up in the middle of the night. They feel like they have tried everything and they are at their wit's end.

You probably figured that once you were past the baby years, waking up at night would be long behind you. But you may find that your little one, or even big one, is *still* getting up at night. Although waking at night is the most common sleep problem of infants and toddlers, it can definitely continue throughout childhood and even into middle school. Studies also indicate that night wakings persist, as children often do not "outgrow" the problem.

Why Does Your Child Wake During the Night?

When it comes to night wakings, the most important thing for parents to understand is that all children, no matter the age, wake briefly throughout the night. These brief wakings, or "arousals," occur between two and six times per night. So the problem is not so much the waking during the night, but rather the fact that your child is unable to return to sleep on her own. When children are able to get themselves right back to sleep after a brief waking during the night, parents are generally blissfully unaware that anything is going on in the room down the hall. In contrast, children who "wake up at night" are those children who can't (or have never learned to) get themselves back to sleep and let their parents know about it in no uncertain terms, either by calling for them or going to their parents' room. Many of these children have developed what we refer to as "negative sleep associations," which makes falling asleep at bedtime and falling back to sleep during the night a problem for both them and you.

What Are Sleep Associations?

Many parents help their child fall asleep by staying with her. They may stay in the child's room until she is asleep or bring her into their own bed. Over time, children learn to rely on this kind of help from their parents in order to fall asleep. Although this may not be a problem at bedtime, it may lead to difficulties with your child falling back to sleep on her own during the night. Thus, sleep associations are conditions that become a habit and are what your child needs in order to fall asleep at bedtime, such as lying next to you. These same sleep associations are then needed in order to fall *back to sleep* during the night. The bottom line is that your child needs to learn to fall asleep on her own so that she can put herself back to sleep when she awakens.

> *Daniel was four years old and fell asleep every night lying down with his mom or dad, while drinking a sippy cup filled with half juice and half water. His parents realized that things had gotten out of hand when every morning they found a line-up of five or six sippy cups next to his bed that they had brought him throughout the night.*

SLEEP ASSOCIATIONS

Sleep associations are things that are present when your child falls asleep and are something that he needs to be able to fall back to sleep when he naturally awakens during the night. A *positive* sleep association helps a child fall asleep on his own, such as cuddling with a stuffed animal, whereas a negative sleep association is something that usually requires reinstatement by a parent during the night. These *negative* sleep associations are the number one cause of frequent wakings during the night.

Why Else Do Children Wake Up at Night?

Obviously, there are lots of reasons why children wake up at night. They may be cold, they may be upset, they may be hungry, they may have had a bad dream, they may have had a bedwetting accident, or any number of other reasons. Your child may also have another sleep disorder, such as sleep apnea (see chapter 13) or periodic limb movement disorder (see chapter 14). Both of these problems can disrupt your child's sleep. Reading about other sleep problems will help you determine a possible cause of your child's nighttime awakenings.

CO-SLEEPING

There are two different kinds of co-sleeping. Some parents wish to share their bed with their child and choose as a family to co-sleep. This is called *lifestyle co-sleeping*. Other families, however, have their child sleep with them in order to try to solve a problem. For example, when your child wakes up at night, it may just be easier to let him sleep with you, or it may be too much of a struggle to get him back in his own bed. This is called *reactive co-sleeping*.

- **Lifestyle co-sleeping.** If you choose to have your child sleep with you, there is no reason to make a change. Eventually, however, as your child gets older, he may wish to sleep in his own room, or *you* may want a change. There is no set age that you must make a change, but most children are typically sleeping in their own bed by the time they start kindergarten or first grade.

- **Reactive co-sleeping.** If this sleeping situation is not working for you or your child, there is no reason that you must keep co-sleeping.

To help your child move from co-sleeping to sleeping on his own, it's often best to do it slowly, especially if he's been sleeping with you for a long time. Start by having your child fall asleep in his own bed while you stay with him. During the night, continue to let him sleep with you. Once your child begins to be comfortable falling asleep in his own room, you can start easing yourself out. Move yourself farther away at bedtime by three to four feet every few nights. Once your child is successful at falling asleep alone at bedtime, then you can start making changes during the night too. For example, he can start spending the entire night in his room, with you there for reassurance. With slow and gradual changes, expect your child to be sleeping on his own within a few weeks.

How Common Is It?

According to a recent poll by the National Sleep Foundation, one-third of parents of preschoolers report that their child wakes at least once per night, and 5 percent wake two or more times. In addition, 14 percent of school-aged children wake up at least one time per night (that parents are aware of). This means that not only are about one out of every eight school-aged children getting up during the night, but they're also letting their parents know about it. Furthermore, just about half (43 percent) of parents of preschool children stay with their child until he is asleep at bedtime, and almost one out of four (23 percent) parents stay with their school-aged child until she drifts off to sleep. Which, when you think about it, suggests that if your child needs you to be there as he falls asleep, there's a 70–80 percent chance he'll need you again at 3:00 AM (ouch!).

Causes

Again, the most common reason for waking up at night is that it has become a learned behavior; your child has come to depend on *you* to fall asleep and fall back to sleep. But don't forget to also think about the multiple other causes of night wakings, such as:

- **Sleep disrupting events.** Anything that disrupts your child's sleep patterns, such as being sick, going on vacation, or a change in schedule, can result in night wakings.
- **Medical problems.** Illness is a common reason for waking at night. Frequent ear infections, pain, asthma, allergies, reflux, and a multitude of other medical problems can disrupt your child's sleep. Be sure to talk with your doctor if you are concerned about any medical problems.
- **Anxiety.** Children who are anxious during the day often are anxious at night as well, leading them to wake up and need reassurance from their parents.
- **Lack of limits.** Your child may be getting up at night because you haven't set clear limits. For example, your child may be allowed to watch television in the middle of the night, or you haven't been consistent in saying *no* to your child coming to your bed at night

(that is, if you don't want him there). Sometimes there is one parent who is much more lax than the other, which can contribute to the problem, as your child knows that Mom or Dad often gives in. It's best (although hard) to have similar rules with both parents.

NAPTIME ISSUES

Many preschoolers still take a nap every day, or need one even if they don't take one. Naptime problems are often the result of the same thing—negative sleep associations. If your child still needs you to lie down with him at naptime, as he does at night, solve bedtime and nighttime issues first and then move on to naptime.

- **Not getting enough sleep.** Surprisingly, not getting enough sleep leads to more wakings at night, not less. So don't stop your child's naps too early if he is still young, get him to bed early, and ensure that he gets enough sleep. If your child is not getting good quality sleep (such as from coughing all night), this can also lead to sleep deprivation and more wakings at night.
- **Stress or change in routine.** Waking up at night can start as a result of something stressful happening in your child's life, such as entering a new school year, or as a result of your child's sleep schedule being disrupted, such as from a trip, jet lag, or illness. This short-term problem, however, can become a long-term one if you're not careful. Staying with your child or spending lots of extra time with him at bedtime and during the night can encourage these wakings and lead to bad sleep habits.

Kim's mother started staying with her at bedtime, because Kim was worried about the start of middle school. Before she knew it, Kim was waking up every night and wanting her mom to stay with her all night.

- **Poor sleep habits.** Waking at night can be the result of other poor sleep habits, such as having an erratic sleep schedule, drinking caffeinated beverages, or doing something too energizing too close to bedtime, such as playing computer games or exercising.

- **Bedroom environment.** Make sure that your child's bedroom is conducive to sleep, that it's not too noisy or too hot, that others do not disrupt his sleep, such as a parent waking up early in the morning to get ready for work or being involved in noisy activities that may disrupt your child's sleep, such as watching television or working on the computer.

Impact of Night Wakings

Waking up at night can cause major problems the next day. For example, your child may be irritable, have more temper tantrums, and have a hard time paying attention in school. He may not do as well at school the following day.

And as we're sure you are well aware, frequent night wakings can result in family stress. With your own sleep disrupted, you may start to feel depressed or anxious, and it can lead to significant marital problems (especially if you don't agree with your partner about how to handle your child's nighttime behavior) and overall stress. Thus, making positive changes in your child's sleep will have major implications across the board—not only will your child sleep better and feel better during the day, but the whole family will sleep better and feel better.

EARLY RISERS

What is too early? For some parents, too early is 5:00 AM, whereas for others it may be 7:00 AM. Realize, though, that younger children usually wake up early in the morning (whereas their teenage counterparts usually wake up too late!). There are basically two groups of children who wake up "too early" in the morning. The first group is those children who have gotten enough sleep and their normal waking time is early in the morning ("larks"). The second group is those who get up for the day before they have really had enough sleep. In this case, the early morning awakening is actually just the final nighttime awakening, but your child can't or won't fall back to sleep for those last few hours. Part of the problem here may be that your child is getting reinforced or rewarded for getting up so early perhaps by being allowed to join you in bed or to watch television while you get a few more minutes sleep.

Ways to Help Your Child Sleep Through the Night

There are a number of things that you can do to help your child sleep through the night:

IT'S NEVER TOO LATE

Even if your child is three, or seven, or even twelve, it's never too late to make changes. You can make a difference, and your child can start sleeping through the night in his own bed.

- **Develop an appropriate sleep schedule with an early bedtime.** Ironically, the more tired your child is, the more times she will awaken during the night (we don't totally know why this happens, but it is likely because your child has more sleep state changes, which, if you remember from chapter 2, can lead to more arousals). So be sure your child continues taking naps during the day (if she is still young), and set an early bedtime. However, that bedtime should be one that is both appropriate for her age (no thirteen-year-old is ever going to go to bed at 8:30) and one that ensures enough sleep at night. Also, having a regular bedtime will set your child's internal clock to be sleepy at the same time every day, helping her to fall asleep more easily.
- **Have a bedtime routine.** Establish a consistent bedtime routine that includes calm and enjoyable activities, such as a bath and bedtime stories. Avoid exciting, high-energy activities, such as playing outside, running around, or watching television. Your child's bedtime routine should consist of three or four soothing activities, such as taking a bath or shower, changing into pajamas, and reading stories. A recent poll by the National Sleep Foundation found that reading stories at bedtime (either being read to or the child reading) was associated with getting more sleep and having fewer sleep problems. Keep it relatively short, though; the whole bedtime routine should last thirty to forty minutes.

- **Keep the bedroom environment consistent.** Make sure that what's going on in your child's bedroom at bedtime (such as having music playing, or having the bedside light on or off) is the same as it will be throughout the night. Remember, if your child always falls asleep to music playing, he may need it turned back on when he wakes up at night.

- **Provide a security object.** Having your child sleep with a security object can help him feel snug and secure in his bed all night. A stuffed animal, a blanket, or having any other type of security object can do the trick (we had a friend whose child slept with an [unopened] tuna fish can; not generally recommended, but, hey, whatever works!).

- **Have your child fall asleep independently.** After the bedtime routine, tuck your child into bed, give a last good-night hug and kiss, and leave the room. Remember, the key to having your child sleep through the night is to have her learn to fall asleep on her own so that she can put herself back to sleep when she naturally awakens during the night.

- **Check on her.** If your child cries or calls for you, check on her periodically. Wait as long or as short a time as you are comfortable with; the exact timing doesn't really matter as long as you're consistent. For some children, checking frequently is effective; for others, checking infrequently works best. Continue returning to check on your child as long as she is crying or upset. The visits should be *brief* (one minute) and *boring; it's sleep time, not playtime!* Calmly tell your child it's time to go to sleep. Remember, the point is to reassure, not to entertain, your child.

- **Respond to your child during the night.** In the beginning, respond to your child throughout the night as you normally would. For example, lying down with him or bringing him into your bed. Research indicates that the majority of children naturally begin sleeping through the night within one or two weeks of falling asleep quickly and easily at bedtime. If your child continues to awaken during the night after several weeks, then use the same checking method during the night as you did at bedtime.

SIX STEPS TO GETTING YOUR CHILD TO SLEEP THROUGH THE NIGHT

Step 1. Establish a set bedtime and regular sleep schedule.

Step 2. Develop a consistent bedtime routine.

Step 3. Make the bedroom environment the same at bedtime as it is throughout the night (e.g., lights, music).

Step 4. Leave your child's room after a last hug and kiss.

Step 5. Check on your child as frequently or infrequently as you wish. The goal is to have your child to fall asleep independently at bedtime.

Step 6. Respond to your child as usual during the night, such as lying down with him. Once your child can fall asleep on his own at bedtime, it his highly likely that within two weeks he will naturally be sleeping through the night. If not, then repeat step 5 with each night waking.

- **Take baby steps.** Some parents feel that not being present when their child falls asleep feels like too big a first step for them and their child. A more gradual approach is to teach your child to fall asleep on her own but with you in the room in the beginning. This approach will take longer, but for some families it feels more comfortable. The first step is to lie down with your child or sit in a chair next to her bed until she is asleep. Once she is able to consistently fall asleep this way, move several feet away every few nights until you are finally in the hallway and no longer in sight.

SUCCESS

In developing a plan to help your child sleep through the night, make sure that it is one in which both you and your child can be successful. You want to set things up so that there is a high likelihood of success. Therefore, it's sometimes better to take smaller steps than a giant leap. For example, if your child always comes into your room during the night and gets in bed with you, start by joining your child in his room when he wakes up. Let him get used to sleeping in his own bed all night before insisting that he not come get you and must fall back to sleep on his own. Thus, small steps that may take up to a few weeks may lead to greater success than a major quick leap that includes too many changes.

- **Return your child to his room during the night.** If your child keeps coming to your room during the night, it's key that you keep returning him to his bed *every single time* it happens (even if it's 3:00 AM and you have an important meeting/plane to catch/big day ahead). If not, your child will keep trying and trying, knowing that eventually you'll cave and he'll be able to stay.

Desiree was six years old and every night came to her parents' room at least once. Most times her parents returned her to her room. However, at least a few nights a week, her parents didn't even wake up when she came in, and they would find her in their bed in the morning. We advised them to do something very simple—hang a bell on a string inside their bedroom door. Whenever Desiree came into their room, the bell rang and woke up her parents. Within a week, Desiree was no longer coming in every night. Sometimes the simplest solution does the trick!

- **Be consistent and don't give up.** The first few nights are likely to be very challenging, and often the second or third night is worse than the first night. Within a few nights to a week, however, you will begin seeing improvement.

STICKER CHARTS AND OTHER REWARDS

Sticker charts are a huge hit with preschoolers and school-aged children. In devising a system, it is most effective if your child gets a reward immediately (e.g., sticker first thing in the morning with an immediate reward) and if there is a high likelihood of his making the goal (e.g., starting off getting a sticker just for sleeping in his own bed all night, even if he calls you often) to reinforce success. With time, you can make the goal more challenging, such as getting a sticker for sleeping in his own bed all night without calling you, and start giving less frequent rewards (e.g., five stickers per week instead of three required to get a reward). If you require your child to go several nights before a reward, don't require consecutive nights, or your child will get frustrated by having to start all over again if he's had a bad night and will be less likely to try again.

Other reward systems can also be very effective. We've sent the sleep fairy to many families' homes, where she leaves a small prize for a good job.

10

"There's a Monster in My Closet": Nighttime Fears and Nightmares

Every night, Timmy's parents have to spend twenty to thirty minutes reassuring him that there are no monsters living in his closet or under his bed. This usually requires them to return to check his room three or four times after they say good-night. Although they want to reassure him, they are frustrated by how long bedtime lasts and how long it takes Timmy to go sleep at night.

Several times a week, four-year-old Deanna wakes up screaming from a frightening dream. Neither she nor her parents can identify anything that may have triggered these dreams, and Deanna has reached the point where she is sometimes scared to fall asleep at night.

Nighttime fears and nightmares are extremely common in children, especially during the preschool years, but they can definitely occur in older children and adolescents as well. They are part of normal development as children's imaginations develop and children begin to understand that there are things that exist that can hurt them. There are times that fears and nightmares are the result of a real-life frightening experience, such as being scared by a large dog or being in a car accident (or even watching the nightly news), but sometimes such fears just seem to come out of the blue.

THE NEWS AND WORLD EVENTS

As children and adolescents get older, they are much more likely to be aware of what is going on in the world, especially as it is portrayed on the news. However, children and adolescents are often not as able to cope with the images that are shown and to understand these events in the context of the world. A seven-year-old may not understand that the earthquake that devastated the South Seas will not affect him living in Nebraska. A nine-year-old may be scared to go to bed after hearing about a child being kidnapped from her bedroom in a city across the country. A fourteen-year-old may keep seeing images in his head of a brutal slaying that was shown over and over again on the news. As you can imagine, such news stories may often lead to fears and nightmares.

So what should you do?

- Talk to your child about what he has heard and what he is feeling.

- Help your child process the news. Talk about these events and what they mean in the context of your child's life.

- Reassure your child that he is safe.

- Monitor your child's exposure to the news, and limit access. Don't keep the news on and repeatedly expose your child to devastating news. It's hard enough to get an image out of your head if you've seen it once. It's impossible if you've seen it ten or twenty times.

- Find a balance between giving your child more information than he can handle and being overprotective and withholding information.

- Stick to family routines as much as possible, as the more familiar things are, the more comforted your child will be.

Nighttime Fears

It's normal for children to have nighttime fears, especially at bedtime, and most children have them at some point. They are part of normal development. These fears usually begin during the preschool years as children develop the cognitive ability to understand that they (or their loved ones) can get hurt or be harmed, or that their loved ones may sometime go away.

NIGHTTIME FEARS

Nighttime fears are very common in preschool children, paralleling cognitive development. Nighttime fears continue throughout childhood and adolescence, but change in their focus. Most fears are usually short-lived, but parents need to differentiate these normal fears from more serious persistent fears, nightmares, and problems with anxiety.

Children typically have different fears at different developmental stages. Young children are often afraid of monsters and other imaginary creatures, whereas older children are more likely to fear being hurt by more realistic dangers, such as burglars or a natural disaster. Oddly enough, young children are usually afraid of things that in real life can't hurt them, like monsters under the bed, but are not afraid of things that actually can, such as leaping off the top of furniture or running out into the middle of a street. It's the job of parents to teach their children what they really need to be afraid of and how to cope with fears.

COMMON FEARS AT DIFFERENT AGES

Age Group	Common Fears
Preschoolers	Being alone
	The dark
	Imaginary creatures
	Monsters
	Animals
	Thunder
	Bodily injury
	Blood
	Needles
School-aged	Threats to self-esteem
	Social situations
	Testing situations
	Bodily injury
	Illness

COMMON FEARS AT DIFFERENT AGES

School-aged *(continued)*	Blood/needles
	Supernatural phenomenon
	(ghosts, witches, aliens)
	Natural disasters
	(earthquakes, hurricanes)
Adolescents	Future events
	The unknown
	Performance failure

What Do Nighttime Fears Look Like?

Obviously, most children look scared when they are afraid. They may cry, cling, and keep leaving their room to be reassured. This can occur at bedtime or in the middle of the night. Some children resist going to bed when they are scared, either refusing to go to bed at all or wanting someone to stay with them. Other children who are anxious insist on sharing a room with a brother or sister or someone else in the house. With older children, the signs may be more subtle and may take the form of multiple requests ("curtain calls") after lights-out (such as a drink of water, another kiss good-night). Resisting going to bed and curtain calls are more common when a child is having difficulty sharing what is bothering him, perhaps because he is embarrassed about being afraid or perhaps because he is just not ready to share his feelings with you.

> *Sarah was nine years old and afraid of the dark. She thought that being scared of the dark was "babyish" and didn't want to tell her parents. Sometimes she pretended to read by flashlight under the covers. She didn't really want to read; it was just reassuring to have the flashlight on.*

> *Gavin was still afraid to sleep alone at age thirteen. He insisted that his four-year-old sister stay in his room with him at night (who was all too*

willing!). He knew that it was ridiculous to expect that a four-year-old would protect him, but it still made him feel better.

Often there are other things that go along with nighttime fears. Some children get so worked up that they have stomachaches or headaches at bedtime or during the night. These pains are real; they are not made up. Many children who are afraid at night are also afraid during the day. They may have the same fears, of being alone or of burglars, or they could be scared of other things.

How Common Is It?

Almost all children have nighttime fears, especially between the ages of three and six years. There is a second peak of nighttime fears in school-aged girls, especially those who are highly anxious during the day.

Causes

Anxiety, stress, and traumatic events can lead to nighttime fears, although the majority of fears can't be linked to any specific event or thing. Family conflict and parental anxiety can also play a role. Anything that makes a child more emotionally aroused is going to make his fears worse and make him feel more anxious. It's one thing to be afraid in the midst of a calm household; it's much easier to be afraid when everything is already tense.

DID SOMETHING TRAUMATIC HAPPEN TO MY CHILD?

Parents often worry that something bad will happen to their child, especially as their child gets older and is spending more and more time away from his parents. Obviously, something stressful or traumatic may indeed affect a child or adolescent and make it more likely that he will be fearful at night and have nightmares. However, these types of events are incredibly rare (despite the coverage they get on the news), and the vast majority of nighttime fears and nightmares are isolated events. If you are worried that something happened to your child, talk to him about whether anything has happened in his life. Check with his teachers and with others who know your child about whether his behavior has changed or whether they know if something is going on.

What Else Could It Be?

Sometimes looking scared at night can be something else. Some other possibilities to consider if your child frequently seems fearful at night are listed below:

- **Bedtime resistance.** Some children learn that saying they are afraid is an effective stalling tactic or a way to avoid bedtime. Understandably, parents are much more sympathetic to being afraid than to refusing to go to bed. This sympathy and attention can encourage your child to continue to be "scared" on subsequent nights. See chapter 8 if you think that your child is simply using being afraid as a ploy to avoid going to bed or going to bed alone.
- **Nightmares.** Some children develop nighttime fears after having a frightening nightmare. They become scared to go to bed or to fall asleep, often avoiding bedtime and falling asleep.
- **Phobias.** Phobias are intense and persistent fears. A child's response to something that they are phobic of is usually quite dramatic, such as running away, appearing terrified, and avoiding what they are afraid of. Some common childhood phobias are fears of snakes, spiders, and dogs. These phobias will also occur during the day and will have an impact on your child's life. For instance, he may avoid going for a hike in the woods because he is phobic of snakes, or he may refuse to go to science class because the teacher may talk about blood or other body parts.
- **Anxiety disorders.** Often in our clinic we see children and adolescents who come in about sleep issues but who actually are suffering from an anxiety disorder. Children and adolescents with anxiety disorders, including generalized anxiety disorder, post-traumatic stress disorder, and separation anxiety disorder, frequently are anxious at bedtime. If your child also worries during the day or is anxious about or avoids certain things, such as going to other children's houses for play dates or being on another floor of the house if no one is with her, then you should consider whether your child has a bigger issue with anxiety than simply bedtime fears.

What to Do When Your Child Is Afraid at Bedtime (or Other Times of the Night)

Dealing with a child who is afraid of the dark or scared to go to bed at night can be like walking a tightrope. It's a fine line between wanting to reassure your child and not wanting to reinforce his fears. If his fears are ignored, your child will not be reassured. If he is reassured too much, you may be subtly giving the message that there is something to be afraid of. Basically, too much reassurance is tacit proof that something scary actually exists or is going to happen. In general, you should be reassuring if your child is younger, while older children typically benefit from an approach that includes teaching and positive reinforcement for independent coping skills. If bedtime fears are affecting your child's ability to fall asleep and stay asleep, try some of the following suggestions:

- **Listen and understand.** Try to understand your child's fears. Don't dismiss or make fun of them, as fears that seem silly to you as an adult may be very real to your child.
- **Be reassuring.** It's important to reassure your child if he is afraid. When your child clings to you as he is being tucked in, or calls out in fear, go back and find out what is wrong. Follow up by saying something like, "You are safe; we are here to make sure you stay safe," or "Mommy and Daddy are right downstairs and we'll always make sure that you are safe." Communicate the idea of safety over and over again.
- **Teach coping skills.** Teach your child coping skills, and discuss alternative ways to respond, such as "being brave" and thinking positive thoughts (e.g., "Monsters are just pretend."). You can also talk about how *you* deal with something that you are afraid of. Also, provide examples of coping role models by reading stories about children who are afraid but conquer their fears.
- **Have fun in the dark.** Make being in the dark fun. Play flashlight tag. Have a treasure hunt and search for things that glow in the dark. Read in the dark by flashlight. Hunt for favorite toys by flashlight in the dark.
- **Use humor.** Teach your child coping skills through the use of

humor. Make a nighttime announcement that "This is Teddy's dad. I declare that this is a safe house. There are no monsters allowed!"

- **Use your imagination and be creative.** Use your imagination to fight imaginary fears like monsters or boogeymen. Many families have found "monster spray" to be a wonderful way to help a child cope with bedtime fears. Take a spray-type water bottle and fill it with water (be sure it has not previously had any chemicals in it, such as plant food). At bedtime, you or your child can spray the room to keep the monsters away. However, it should be noted that some young children view this as evidence that a monster actually exists! In addition to monster spray, there are other ways you can be creative and help your child. For example, consider allowing her to have a pet for nighttime company. Even a bedside fish tank may help. Whenever possible, actively involve your child in coming up with solutions to help him gain a sense of mastery and control.

MAGIC MOMMY BUBBLE

One mom has a bedtime ritual that she has done every night since her children were small: keeping them safe in a "magic mommy bubble" throughout the night. While touching each body part with both her hands, encasing them in a bubble with her touch, she sings to them, "Your head and shoulders and arms and chest and belly and legs and knees and wiggly-wiggly toes." At ages ten and seven, her boys still request their magic mommy bubble every night. She even sings it to them at bedtime over the phone when she is out of town.

- **Provide a security object.** Help your child become attached to a security object that he can keep in bed with him. This can help him feel more relaxed at bedtime and throughout the night. Even older children and teens (and some adults, for that matter) feel better with a cuddly stuffed critter nearby.
- **Use a nightlight.** No matter what your child seems to be afraid of, a nightlight can help. Nightlights are fine as long as they don't prevent your child from falling asleep. Another thing to try is leaving

the bedroom door open so that your child doesn't feel isolated from the rest of the family.

- **Avoid scary television shows/movies/video games.** Keep your child away from scary TV shows, videos, or stories that may add to his fears.
- **Relax.** Teach your child relaxation strategies to help him relax at bedtime and fall asleep. This will give him something else to think about while lying in bed and will help distract him from his fearful thoughts. Also, it is physically impossible to be relaxed and scared at the same time.
- **Discuss your child's fears during the day.** Talk with your child about his fears during the day and how he can be less frightened at night. Additionally, build your child's self-confidence during the day. If he feels secure during the day, this can help him feel more secure at night, too.
- **Set limits.** At the same time that you are reassuring your child, you do need to set limits. Setting limits is necessary to prevent your child's "being scared" behavior from being reinforced. Checking closets and leaving a low nightlight on are reasonable, but starting to sleep with your child every night may not be. Also, encourage appropriate behavior, such as reminding your child, "Remember, no crying and no calling out at bedtime."
- **Keep him in bed.** Don't encourage your child to get out of bed. He should stay in bed and find out for himself that he really is safe so that he can learn to overcome his fears. If you bring your child into your room, or allow him to come downstairs while you finish the dinner dishes, the message is that his bed isn't a safe place to be. It is much better for you to stay with him in his room than it is for him to join you. If your child is too frightened to stay in *his* room alone, it is okay to *occasionally* stay with him until he falls asleep. Don't do this too frequently, or even two nights in a row, as he may come to depend on your presence. Similarly, if your child wakes up in the middle of the night and can't go back to sleep because he is frightened, go and reassure him. Repeat the message about being safe and that he will be fine. If your child gets up in the middle of

the night and comes into your room, it is better to take him right back and gently tuck him into bed. Again reassure him, and let him know that he will be okay.

• **Check on him.** If your child is anxious about you leaving, check on him frequently. Begin by briefly checking and reassuring him in five minutes, and then every ten minutes until he is asleep. It is better to check on him on a predictable schedule, every five or ten minutes, so that your coming in and reassuring him is not based on him crying or calling out for you.

• **Reach for the stars.** Sometimes parents inadvertently reinforce a child for being scared at night by giving him lots of attention for being afraid. If this is the case, switch the scenario. Give your son lots of attention for dealing with his fears. Tell him how proud you are of him for being brave. Set up a star system so he can earn stars for being brave and sleeping on his own. Be as specific as possible about what he needs to do (staying in bed all night, not calling out after lights-out). Also, the reward schedule should be set up so that there is a high likelihood of being successful (e.g., a nightly rather than just a weekly reward, at least at the beginning). In addition, after earning a certain number of stars, allow him to turn them in for a treat, such as watching a favorite video, going to the park, or baking chocolate chip cookies.

• **Be on the alert for severe or persistent anxiety.** If your child's anxiety and fears continue, are severe, or are also present during the day, consider taking him for a psychological evaluation to identify and treat anxiety.

Nightmares

Nightmares are scary dreams that can wake a child, leaving her upset and in need of comfort. They are practically universal in childhood. It is rare to find someone who has never experienced a nightmare. After a nightmare, most children are afraid to go back to sleep and often do not want to be left alone. Very young children don't know the difference between a dream and reality, so when they wake up they may not understand the concept that they were only dreaming and it is now over. They may keep insisting that something scary is still about to occur.

What do children have nightmares about? Most young toddlers have concerns about being separated from their parents. So they may have a nightmare about being lost or something happening to one of their parents. Nightmares also are more likely to occur following some difficult or stressful event in the child's life. For example, if a child has just started a new school or is away from home overnight, she is more likely to have a nightmare. Nightmares may also be the reliving of a traumatic event, such as getting lost or being bit by a dog. Older children often have nightmares related to scary movies or stories or a frightening daytime experience.

NIGHTMARES

Nightmares are frightening dreams from which a child wakes up and usually needs comforting.

How Common Is It?

Studies indicate that about 75 percent of children report having had at least one nightmare, and up to 50 percent of young children have had a nightmare that results in their needing their parents during the night. One study of *chronic nightmares,* defined as having frequent nightmares for at least three months, found that 24 percent of children ages two to five and 41 percent of six- to ten-year-olds experienced this as an ongoing issue.

Causes

Just like nighttime fears, nightmares are usually a part of normal development and are a sign of a child's developing imagination. Children are also more likely to have nightmares after a frightening or stressful experience. Children who are anxious in general are more likely to have frequent and more intense nightmares. Surprisingly, not getting enough sleep can lead to intense and vivid dreams, including nightmares. In this situation, sleep deprivation leads to an increase in REM sleep, or "dream sleep," the stage of sleep in which nightmares occur. By the same token, there are some medications (some antidepressants, antihistamines, and caffeine, for example) that decrease REM sleep when you are taking them and increase REM sleep when you stop ("REM rebound"), which can lead to more nightmares.

Ben has always been more anxious than other children his age, always worrying about his schoolwork and not wanting to play at other children's houses. Not only does he worry more than other kids, but he also seems to have many more nightmares than other kids his age. His parents don't recall his two older brothers having nightmares as often as Ben does.

Ways to Reduce the Likelihood That Your Child Will Have a Nightmare

- **Avoid scary things before bedtime.** Don't read scary stories or watch scary movies or television shows immediately before bedtime. Choose instead a comforting bedtime routine.
- **Minimize stress.** If there is something in your child's life that you know is distressing, try to take care of it and reassure your child. If your child suddenly starts having lots of nightmares, try to figure out why. Look for recurring themes that could give you a clue as to the cause.
- **Make sure your child is getting enough sleep.** Children are much more likely to have nightmares after not getting enough sleep. So if your child is having nightmares, make sure that she is getting enough sleep, as this can help decrease both of the number of nightmares and their intensity.

Additional Issues

Many children who have nightmares also have daytime or nighttime fears. Also, some children may start to resist going to bed at night. They begin to associate going to bed and bedtime with having scary dreams, and so wish to avoid it. Don't be surprised if your child does this.

Lucinda, a nine-year-old, began having nightmares of car crashes and being chased by dead relatives after driving by a particularly gruesome-looking car accident on the highway. For several weeks, she had nightmares almost every night. She became scared to go to bed, as she didn't want to fall asleep and have another awful nightmare.

What Else Could It Be?

Most of the time, parents can tell when their child has a nightmare. It's usually quite obvious. But there are other times when your child may appear awake and frightened during the night. It is important to differentiate these times from nightmares:

- **Sleep terrors.** Parents often have a difficult time distinguishing between nightmares and sleep terrors. Nightmares, in comparison to sleep terrors (see chart in chapter 12), usually occur in the second half of the night, when most REM sleep occurs. In addition, your child will be able to tell you all about the scary dream that he had and will remember the entire thing the next morning. However, with a sleep terror, which usually occurs in the first few hours of the night, your child will not be able to tell you about a specific detailed dream, other than maybe just a feeling of being scared, and will not remember it the next morning. After a nightmare, your child may have a hard time falling back to sleep, whereas sleep terrors end abruptly, with your child returning quickly to deep sleep. Also, your child will be confused during a sleep terror, but not after a nightmare. (For more information on sleep terrors, see chapter 12.)

WHO IS MORE UPSET THE NEXT MORNING?

If your child is more upset the next morning, it was a nightmare. If you are more upset, it's most likely a sleep terror.

- **Psychiatric problems.** Frequent nightmares can be associated with emotional and psychiatric problems, including anxiety disorders, bipolar disorder, and schizophrenia. If your child is having emotional and psychological problems during the day, be sure to seek out help, whether from your child's doctor or from a psychologist or psychiatrist. A school psychologist can also be a good resource.

How Should You Respond to Your Child's Nightmares?

In general, when your child is young, he will need you to reassure him after a nightmare. However, as your child gets older, you will want to start teaching him coping skills that he himself can use when he is anxious or scared.

- **Be reassuring.** The best thing that you can do if your child has a nightmare is to comfort her. Following most nightmares, your child will be reassured by a few minutes of comfort. Stay with her in her room. Let her know that you are nearby and will make sure that she is safe and secure. Most children are still tired after a nightmare and will be ready to fall back to sleep.
- **Provide a security object.** Help your child become attached to a security object that he can keep in bed with him. This can help him feel more relaxed and safe throughout the night. A family pet that stays in your child's bedroom, whether it's the family cat or even a goldfish, can also be reassuring.
- **Leave a light on.** If your child insists on you turning a light on and leaving it on, that is okay. If you leave it on, put it on the dimmest setting possible so that your child can fall back to sleep.
- **Discuss it the next day.** The next day, you may want to try talking to your child about her nightmare to see if there is anything bothering her. Most of the time, nightmares are isolated events with little meaning, but if your child starts having them on a frequent basis, it is best to try to figure out what is disturbing her.
- **Use your (and her) imagination.** Some children do well with using their imagination to get rid of nightmares. A child can draw pictures of their bad dreams and throw them away, or they can imagine different endings to their nightmares. A dream catcher hung over a child's bed can be reassuring. According to Native American tradition, the hole in the middle of the dream catcher lets good dreams pass through, and the web catches bad dreams. You can also suggest that your child pretend he's watching a television and can "change the channel" in his mind to move to a new dream. Or have him flip his pillow over for a fresh start.
- **Relax.** Relaxation techniques can help a child relax at bedtime and after having a bad dream. There are many different kinds of relaxation strategies, including meditation and guided imagery. Guided imagery involves having your child imagine a relaxing scene, such as being on the beach or watching a sunset. Help him use all of his senses during guided imagery, such as smelling the salt air, hearing

the seagulls squawk, feeling the heat of the sun and the sand in his hands, and seeing the waves crash on the beach. There are also some excellent relaxation tapes available that your child can listen to. You can purchase relaxation tapes can through the Anxiety Disorders Association of America (ADAA; www.adaa.org) or the Child Anxiety Network (www.childanxiety.net).

- **Take it slow.** Systematic desensitization is a more sophisticated technique that combines relaxation strategies with gradual exposure to a particular thing that is scaring your child. It is often used to help people deal with phobias. To start, help your child learn to relax. Next, with your child, develop a series of activities or thoughts that go from the least scary to the most frightening. For example, if your child is afraid of dogs, the series might look like this: (1) looking at a picture of a dog, (2) watching a friend play with a puppy, (3) petting a cute puppy, (4) being near a medium-sized friendly dog, and (5) being near a large dog. Starting with the least frightening (looking at a picture) helps your child pair these activities or thoughts with being relaxed, so that he begins to associate the thought or activity with feeling calm and collected instead of anxious and scared. As your child masters each step (stops being scared when he looks at a picture of a dog), you can move on to the next level (petting a dog), and so on. This technique can be particularly helpful with nightmares that have a recurrent theme.

11

Tossing and Turning: Insomnia

Every night is frustrating for twelve-year-old Patricia and her parents. Starting at around 8.00, Patricia becomes increasingly upset and worries that she won't be able to fall asleep. Her parents have tried talking to her, but the more suggestions they make, the more upset Patricia becomes. They have also tried encouraging her to relax, to take a soothing bath, to drink warm milk, and to write down her concerns. There have been many nights when they end up yelling at Patricia to "just go to bed."

Insomnia can be defined, fairly simply, as difficulty falling asleep or staying asleep. Insomnia can be a short-term problem of difficulty falling asleep for just a night or two in conjunction with a stressful event, or it can be a long-term struggle to get some shut-eye, lasting months to years. It's important to understand that insomnia is a *symptom*, with as many possible causes as there are sheep to count. Just like pain, which can be a symptom of many different things, insomnia can be the result of another sleep disorder; a psychological problem, such as anxiety; medication; a medical disorder; or just about any condition you can name that interferes with sleep. When the insomnia appears to develop relatively out of the blue and does not seem related to anything else, it's usually known as *primary insomnia*. This is the type of insomnia we cover in this chapter. Most of the time, primary insomnia is a combination of emotional (worry, stress) and physical (increased muscle tension) factors that we call *psychophysiological insomnia*. It's also known as *learned* or *behavioral insomnia*. Although it is one of the most common sleep complaints in adults, this type of insomnia is much less frequent in children and adolescents.

"You mean people learn how *not* to fall asleep?" You bet. You see, insomnia is almost always the result of learned poor sleep habits (such as spending too much time in bed, napping during the day, and not going to bed and waking up at the same time every day), as well as learned negative thoughts about sleep, such as "I'll never be able to fall asleep tonight (or probably for the rest of my life)."

> *Diana, a fifteen-year-old, has been having problems sleeping for the past two years, ever since she started high school. She worries throughout the day that she won't be able to fall asleep and will then be too tired to concentrate in school. She has always been an A student, but recently her grades have been slipping. Diana is also involved in many after-school activities. When she gets home from school or sports practice, she starts worrying about how she will sleep that night. Diana often takes a nap when she gets home around 5:00, because she feels that's the only time she can get some sleep.*

INSOMNIA

Insomnia involves difficulty falling asleep, staying asleep, or waking too early in the morning. In many cases, insomnia is a symptom of another sleep disorder or medical disorder. Insomnia as a disorder involves poor sleep habits and negative thoughts about sleep.

How Common Is It?

We don't really know exactly how many school-aged children or adolescents have insomnia. However, several studies have found that 12 to 33 percent of adolescents state that they are "poor sleepers."

Studies of adults have consistently found that insomnia is more common in women than in men. There is some evidence to suggest that it is also more common in adolescent girls than in boys. However, some part of this difference may be due to a reporting bias, which means that girls and women may be more likely to *admit* that they have a problem (and seek help for it) than men and boys are (let's just say this isn't surprising and leave it at that).

Causes

Primary insomnia is almost always the result of some combination of the following factors:

- **Bad sleep habits.** Children and adolescents with insomnia very often have very poor sleep habits, such as going to bed at irregular hours and lying in bed for hours trying to fall asleep.
- **Negative thoughts about sleep.** Negative thoughts, beliefs, and attitudes about sleep are common; such as: "If I don't fall asleep right now, I won't be able to get in the morning. If I can't get up, I'll miss my history exam. If I miss my history exam, I'll get an F for the quarter, and if I do that, I won't get into a decent college and make something of myself. Okay, I'm doomed." This kind of distorted view of the dire consequences of the sleep problem sounds ridiculous in the cold light of day, of course, but is very common among insomniacs. It's also what helps keep the whole "worry–can't sleep–worry even more–sleep even less–*really* start to worry" cycle going.
- **Sleeping in.** It may surprise you to learn that one of the most common mistakes that people with insomnia make is spending *too much time* in bed. For one thing, lying in bed for hours trying to fall asleep just sets you up to associate being in bed with being *awake* (and worrying about it) instead of being asleep! Some insomniacs overestimate how much sleep they actually need, and get frustrated when they can't fall asleep at an unrealistically early hour. Others sleep in on weekends to catch up on sleep lost during the week, which results in not being tired enough to fall asleep again the next night.
- **The Three *P*s.** Insomnia in most people results from a combination of *predisposing* factors, which make a person more likely to develop insomnia (such as inheriting a tendency for insomnia); *precipitating* factors (like starting a new school, breaking up with a boyfriend); and *perpetuating* factors (such as poor sleep habits, caffeine use, and those doom-and-gloom thoughts about sleep). This basically means that for any given child or adolescent to develop insomnia, she must be vulnerable to developing it in the first place. Just as some children are more likely to get headaches or stomachaches, other children

have a higher likelihood of developing insomnia. This predisposition may be genetic. There do seem to be some families in which several generations all have difficulty sleeping. Or it may be a personality trait (insomniacs tend to be worrywarts). In those who are predisposed to having insomnia, the onset of sleep difficulties is often triggered by an event or situation such as going back to school after the summer, an illness, or increased stress at school. Once the insomnia ball gets rolling, however, it's kept in motion by those perpetuating behaviors, which, ironically, are often the very things that insomniacs do thinking they will *help* the insomnia (like taking naps or lying in bed for hours trying to fall asleep)!

Stephen began having insomnia when he was twelve years old. It began after he started a new school. Six months later, though, he is still having a hard time falling asleep. Most nights, he lies in bed tossing and turning for an hour or two. His mother tries to help him settle down, but Stephen always ends up frustrated. On some mornings, his mother has given him a small cup of coffee to help him wake up for school. Several times a week, Stephen takes a nap before starting his homework. Both Stephen and his parents are frustrated and can't figure out how to solve his sleep problems.

The Fourth *P*: Personality. Adolescents with primary insomnia tend to be anxious, and are often perfectionists and academic overachievers. This may lead to a vicious cycle in which they get very anxious about how the insomnia is going to affect their school performance, which then leads to even more difficulty falling asleep.

INSOMNIA MAY PREDICT LATER DEPRESSION

In some children and adolescents, insomnia and problems sleeping can predict depression later on. It can be a sign of the development of depression. So if your child has insomnia, especially if he had always been a good sleeper, be sure to watch out for other symptoms of depression. Other symptoms of depression include sadness, changes in appetite, social withdrawal (not wanting to be with friends), lack of enjoyment in favorite activities, and thoughts of hurting oneself. Talk with your child's doctor if you think your child may be depressed.

Clues

Here are some clues to look for that suggest your child or adolescent may have insomnia:

- **Sleep problems.** Your child or adolescent with insomnia will have difficulty falling asleep, staying asleep, or sometimes waking too early in the morning (this can be a sign of depression as well).
- **Behaviors that interfere with sleep.** These behaviors may include such things as worrying during the day that she won't be able to sleep that night and trying too hard to fall asleep in bed. But here's the thing—adolescents with insomnia usually can fall asleep easily at other times, such as while watching television, or in other locations, like a friend's house or a hotel. That's because they don't associate those other situations with their sleep problems. It just goes to show you the power of mind over matter!
- **Anxiety about sleep.** Your child or adolescent may be tense and worried about going to bed and about being able to sleep. For some kids, this anxiety starts as soon as dinner is over, continues to build throughout the evening, and is full-blown by the time lights-out occurs.
- **Daytime problems.** Your child or adolescent may complain that she has a hard time dragging herself out of bed in the morning and functioning during the day.

Other possible insomnia clues include:

- **Changes in mood.** Children and adolescents with insomnia may be moody, irritable, and all-around difficult to live with.
- **Daytime fatigue.** Children and adolescents with insomnia often feel fatigued and blah during the day and have little energy, but are rarely actually sleepy.
- **Poor school performance.** Some children and adolescents may have problems in school, which is often related to the fatigue and low energy.
- **Empty Coke cans in the back seat.** To keep themselves awake and fight fatigue, many adolescents with sleep problems down caf-

feinated beverages all day long (see chapter 5 for more of the skinny on caffeine). But of course the more caffeine they drink during the day, the more difficult it is for them to fall asleep at night, keeping the whole cycle in motion.

- **Taking sleeping pills (or worse).** Taking prescription or over-the-counter sleeping medications is common in adults with insomnia, but adolescents and college-aged students may also use over-the-counter medications like Benadryl or Tylenol PM to curb those sleepless nights. Adolescents, like adults, have also been known to use a beer or two to help themselves fall asleep. This is a very bad idea for a multitude of reasons, not the least of which is that alcohol helps you doze off initially, but keeps you awake once its effect wears off in the middle of the night.

Making the Diagnosis

There is no "test" for insomnia, so the diagnosis is made based on the description of the sleep problem and on making sure, by process of elimination, that there are no other underlying causes of the insomnia symptoms that need to be treated or addressed. This means that a careful review of details like your child's medical history, emotional state, and other sleep issues is necessary. It's important to make sure that the insomnia is not actually due to another problem, such as another sleep disorder, a medical disorder, or a psychiatric problem. Since you as a parent can't really do that yourself, it's best to consult your child's doctor about her insomnia problem.

But your input is invaluable. For example, having you and/or your child with insomnia keep a sleep diary or log can be very helpful in ruling out other problems, teasing out the specifics, and coming up with a treatment plan. (Sample sleep diaries are provided in appendix A.) A two-week sleep diary can yield detailed and valuable information about how often your child has trouble sleeping, on what nights of the week, and if there are any identifiable patterns to the sleeping difficulties. It also helps to point out sleep behaviors that may be counterproductive and may be making the insomnia worse (like taking catnaps during the day). Sometimes a sleep diary may reveal that the "insomniac" is actually sleeping more or better than she thinks she is. Remember, it's very common for people with insomnia to worry excessively and blow things out of proportion when it comes to sleep.

Courtney kept a sleep diary for two weeks. She had been complaining about not being able to sleep for several months. When she and her mother sat down and looked at her sleep diaries, they noticed that Courtney had the most trouble sleeping on Tuesday and Thursday nights. They realized those were the nights she had basketball practice. On the way to practice, the family usually went by a fast-food restaurant to pick up a quick dinner. Courtney always got a caffeinated soda, and those were the only times she had caffeine so late in the day. Once Courtney changed drinks, she found that she slept much better.

Bethany (a sixteen year old), who tends to be somewhat of a perfectionist, was terribly worried about her sleep and claimed that she "never sleeps more than two to three hours a night." However, in reviewing her two-week sleep log, she was actually getting more like six or seven hours on a fairly regular basis. Although that's still short of what she needs, she was relieved to see that the problem was not as bad as she had thought, and felt much less frantic about fixing the problem right away.

Although generally not necessary in evaluating a child with insomnia, there are situations in which your child's doctor may want to order some tests. For example, blood work may be requested to check for iron deficiency anemia (particularly common in teenage girls) or a low thyroid level, especially if your child is very fatigued during the day. An overnight sleep study is rarely done when evaluating for insomnia, unless your doctor suspects another sleep disorder, such as sleep apnea (see chapter 13) or periodic limb movement disorder (see chapter 14).

What Else Could It Be?

Insomnia, as discussed above, is a symptom that can be the result of a number of sleep disorders or other factors. It is crucial to try to figure out if there are any other causes of your child's insomnia.

- **Transient insomnia.** *Transient,* or short-term, insomnia typically occurs in people who have always slept well in the past. Transient insomnia can be the result of sleeping somewhere unfamiliar, such as at camp, or somewhere that is not conducive to sleep, such as somewhere that is too hot or too noisy. A trip, jet lag, being sick, or a stressful event can all disrupt sleep too.

- **Restless legs syndrome.** A child or adolescent with a sleep problem called *restless legs syndrome* (RLS) (see chapter 14) will also have difficulty falling asleep at bedtime. However, what prevents the child or adolescent with RLS from falling asleep is an uncomfortable ("creepy-crawly") feeling in the legs that gets worse when lying still and gets better with moving the legs around. Because most kids (and many adults) with RLS don't know enough about the disorder to complain about these symptoms, it's important to ask your child directly (especially if this condition runs in your family).

- **Delayed sleep phase syndrome.** Delayed sleep phase syndrome (see chapter 15) is a fairly common sleep disorder in adolescents and can look a lot like insomnia. Teenagers with a delayed sleep phase typically aren't physically ready to fall asleep until one, two, or three o'clock in the morning. So if they try to fall asleep at, say, 11:00 PM, the result is several hours of watching the clock and staring at the ceiling before finally conking out. However, the teenager with delayed sleep phase will fall asleep pronto if he goes to bed at his preferred bedtime (2:00 AM). In contrast, adolescents with insomnia complain of problems falling asleep no matter what time they go to bed. In addition, adolescents with delayed sleep phase syndrome when allowed to choose their own sleep schedule (like during the summer or once they go to college), fall asleep and wake up at about the same time (late) every day and their sleep "problem" magically disappears.

- **Psychiatric disorders.** Insomnia often goes hand in hand with depression and anxiety, and it is sometimes difficult to figure out which came first. Kids who are depressed usually have other related symptoms, such as loss of appetite and feelings of worthlessness or hopelessness. They may also be withdrawn and sad. Generally, kids with anxiety disorders are anxious about many things, not just about being able to sleep at night, and are anxious *all* the time, both during the day and at night.

- **Medical issues.** Difficulty falling asleep may be the result of a medical disorder, such as asthma, allergies, and headaches, as well as other medical conditions, such as pain or physical discomfort (see chapter 19 for a review of sleep and medical disorders). Certain medications can also interfere with sleep, especially stimulants used for ADHD (see chapter 17).

Sleep Solutions

Insomnia, because it is a learned habit, requires effort and patience to treat. Some possible things that you can try include the following:

- **Clean up your child's sleep.** Although adopting what we sleep experts call "good sleep hygiene" alone is unlikely to completely solve an insomnia problem, getting rid of old bad sleep habits and developing new good ones is essential for children and adolescents with insomnia. Good sleep habits include (1) keeping a regular sleep schedule (going to bed and waking up at the same time every day), (2) avoiding caffeine, tobacco, and other drugs, (3) sleeping in a bedroom that is cool, quiet, and comfortable, (4) developing a bedtime routine that is calming and sleep-friendly, and (5) avoiding stimulating activities just before bed, like playing computer games and watching television. (See chapter 3 for more information on age-appropriate, sleep-friendly habits for your child.)
- **Relax.** Helping your child or adolescent learn relaxation strategies, such as deep breathing, positive mental imagery (picturing herself on an endless expanse of sun-drenched beach), or meditation, can help her relax her mind and body at bedtime and fall asleep. This has the added benefit of giving her something constructive to do instead of lying in bed, thinking about not being able to fall asleep.
- **Get a new attitude.** Since most children or adolescents with insomnia have negative thoughts about sleep and sleeping, these thoughts need to be replaced by positive ones. For example, rather than saying, "I'll never be able to get to sleep tonight," it is better to think, "You know what, I'll just relax and rest at bed-

time tonight." Try substituting "If I don't fall asleep, it will be a complete disaster" with "Well, the worst that can happen is that I'll be a little tired in the morning."

- **Don't be a clock-watcher.** Remove the clock from your child's bedroom, as watching the clock tick away the sleepless hours just causes more stress and makes it all that much more difficult to fall asleep.
- **Get out of bed.** Remember the association many people with insomnia have between being in bed and being awake? Rather than lying in bed tossing and turning, it's far better to have your child or adolescent get out of bed and *do something else* to help reverse this association between bed and sleeplessness. If he can't fall asleep after twenty minutes or so (an estimate, since the clock is out of the room, right?), he should get out of bed and do something that is relaxing but boring, such as reading a magazine or listening to music (*not* watching television). The idea is not to get involved in something fun that will keep him up. When he feels drowsy, only then should he get back in bed and try to fall asleep. If sleep remains elusive for another twenty minutes, repeat the process. As many times as it takes. Warning: this is a *lot* harder than it sounds and is probably the single biggest reason that people with insomnia give up on behavioral treatment. But it's a key point in getting better.
- **Restrict time in bed.** The same basic principle of reversing those bad bed-sleep associations applies here. Temporarily set your child's bedtime later so that the *time she spends in bed* is approximately equal to the *amount of time she is actually sleeping* (with a lower limit of five to six hours). This means you need to subtract any time she is in bed at bedtime or during the night trying unsuccessfully to sleep. Since this amount of sleep is probably not enough, she is more likely to be sleepy the next day. And being extra sleepy has the additional perk of helping your child or adolescent fall asleep more quickly and stay asleep the next night and so on. Once she is falling asleep at the later bedtime within twenty minutes or so, you can start moving her bedtime earlier by fifteen

minutes every few nights until you're back to her normal bedtime. Warning: since this strategy usually involves some degree of sleep deprivation, it's not a good idea to try it at a time when your child otherwise really needs to be alert (like during exams).

- **Use the bed for sleeping.** Hmmm, that sounds like a no-brainer. But teenagers in particular are likely to use their bed as a kind of "command central," doing everything on it from homework to talking on the phone to plotting their latest strategy for getting you to give them a later curfew. For most teens, this is no problem. But for the insomniac teen, this just reinforces that old association of bed = wide-awake. So move the activities elsewhere and use the bed for counting sheep.

Fourteen-year-old Jenna had been having problems falling asleep for the past few years. She went to bed at 10:00 PM, but would then toss and turn until she eventually fell asleep at 12:30. She began by making changes to her sleep schedule, being sure to not sleep in too much on weekends and turning off her radio at bedtime. She also moved her bedtime to 12:00, and did a relaxation exercise to help her fall asleep. In just a week, she was falling asleep within twenty minutes of getting in bed. She than started to slowly move her bedtime earlier by fifteen minutes. This ended up being more difficult than she expected. Every time she moved her bedtime earlier, it took longer to fall asleep. She had hoped that she would be able to move her bedtime back to 10:00 quickly, but it ended up taking about six weeks, with her making very gradual changes instead.

12

Things That Go Bump in the Night: Sleepwalking and Sleep Terrors

"Every night around 10:30 Billy bolts out of bed and starts screaming uncontrollably. I often find him running around his room looking frantic. I try to hold him, but he just pushes me away and looks terrified. I don't understand it, and it frightens me."

"Yesterday morning I found Sarah asleep in the downstairs closet. She says she has no idea how she got there. And last month, she tried to get out the front door at three in the morning. It's lucky I caught her!"

No, strange as it seems, Billy's behavior, described above, is not evidence that he is "possessed," and his mom is decidedly not crazy. Billy has sleep terrors. And Sarah is not trying to run away from home in the middle of the night; she is sleepwalking. These kinds of unusual behaviors that occur during the night are what sleep experts call *parasomnias*. Although they are basically harmless, it can understandably be quite a frightening experience for you as a parent to see your child in the midst of a sleep terror, or to awaken in the middle of the night to find your child has sleepwalked his way over to your bed.

Sleepwalking is very common in children. Children who are sleepwalking may wander around the house, actually leave the house (including through locked doors), or just head to the bathroom. A sleepwalking child generally has his eyes open, usually appears confused or dazed during an episode, and may mumble and give odd or incoherent answers to questions.

When your child walks in his sleep, he may be clumsy and may even do bizarre or strange things, like urinating in a closet. Some children walk in their sleep every night, while others only do it once throughout their childhood. You may not even know that your child has walked in his sleep if he just gets up, wanders around a bit, and then goes back to his room for the rest of the night.

SLEEPWALKING

Sleepwalking is common in children, usually occurring during the first few hours of the night.

Sleep terrors, on the other hand, would be hard to miss. Not called "terrors" for nothing, these nighttime episodes are much more dramatic and can be distressing to watch. During a sleep terror your child may appear very agitated, frightened, and even panicked. He may appear confused and dazed. He may cry out, scream, mumble, and give weird answers to questions. Your child may flail about, push you away, or behave in other strange ways. In addition, during these events your child may avoid being comforted. He may actually get more upset if you try to calm him down or wake him up. This can be the most difficult part for parents. In fact, sleep terrors are much worse to witness than to experience. For your child, a sleep terror is not upsetting like a typical nightmare or bad dream would be. As disturbing and frightening as these events may appear to you, your child is blissfully unaware of what he is doing. And while you're still shaking the next morning, he will have absolutely no memory of any of the goings-on the next day.

Although your sleepwalker or your child in the middle of a sleep terror may appear awake, his brain is actually in the deepest stage of sleep. That's why he doesn't remember anything the next morning and why he seems to look right through you when you call his name. It's also why he may fall down the stairs or walk into a wall while sleepwalking. He is basically stuck halfway between asleep and awake. Since deep or slow wave sleep is concentrated at the beginning of the night, that's the time when both sleep terrors and sleepwalking tend to (but not always) occur. All of this distinguishes sleep terrors and sleepwalking from nightmares, which occur during "dream" (REM) sleep and often awaken a child from sleep. Although it may look like it, your child is not dreaming during these events. Sleep terrors are also not a sign of some deep-seated psychological problem or the result of a traumatic event. As bizarre as they appear, sleep terrors and sleepwalking are really normal developmental events that almost always disappear as a child gets older, his brain matures, and the percent of his sleep that is deep sleep drops dramatically during adolescence.

SLEEP TERRORS

Sleep terrors are a sudden arousal from deep sleep, with a child looking upset and frightened.

COMMON CHARACTERISTICS OF SLEEPWALKING AND SLEEP TERRORS

- Usually occurs during the first few hours of the night (can also occur during naps)
- Episodes can last from a few minutes to an hour
- Child is agitated and confused
- Child avoids comfort
- Child does not remember the event the next day
- Ends quickly with a child falling back into a deep sleep
- Does not involve dreaming
- Exacerbated by sleep deprivation or an underlying sleep disrupter

---

Clues

Sleepwalking and sleep terror episodes usually occur in the first few hours after falling asleep, and last a few minutes to a half-hour. Some children have them only once in their lifetime, whereas others have them every night. Some children even have multiple episodes in a single night. One memorable five-year-old who came to our sleep clinic a number of years ago was literally experiencing as many as fifty to sixty brief night terrors (documented in the sleep lab) a night. While her exhausted parents were reeling the next morning from staying up all night with a highly agitated child, our kindergartener was up at 6:00 every day, full of beans and ready to tackle the day, with no clue whatsoever as to what all the fuss was about!

- **Little wanderers.** Parents are generally able to tell that their child is sleepwalking, although it is not always obvious that your child is actually asleep. Sometimes the only way to tell that your child is sleepwalking is that she does something unusual or bizarre, such as going into a brother or sister's room in the middle of the night or wandering into a closet.

Sondra was very upset with her eleven-year-old daughter, Michaela, for getting up in the middle of the night and making herself a snack. Michaela vehemently denied doing it, which made her mother even angrier, as she thought Michaela was also lying. It ended up that Michaela was sleepwalking and had no recollection of these events.

RISK OF INJURY

Your child can get hurt when sleepwalking or during a sleep terror. He can fall down the stairs, try to climb out a window, or walk out into traffic. Be sure that you keep your child safe—lock all outside doors, secure windows, and don't leave sharp or dangerous objects lying around.

- **Holy terrors.** Sleep terrors usually start suddenly with your child appearing peacefully asleep one minute then appearing extremely upset, frightened, and confused the next. She may hyperventilate, her heart may be pounding, she may be sweating, and her pupils may be dilated. Your child may be clumsy and may flail, push you away, or behave in other strange ways. Sleep terrors, however, may be much milder (sometimes described as a *confessional arousal*), and your child may simply appear somewhat agitated and confused.

Other things that may go along with sleepwalking and sleep terrors:

- **Slumber party slump.** Because of the potential embarrassment and safety issues, many children and adolescents who sleepwalk or have sleep terrors avoid social situations such as sleepovers or overnight summer camp.
- **Parental anxiety.** Because of the unusual nature of these events, parents are often understandably very anxious about whether there is an underlying meaning to these episodes and how to respond to them. They are often concerned about not being present during one of the episodes, so they tend to avoid using babysitters and may think twice about taking that weekend getaway.

How Common Is It?

Between 15 percent and 40 percent of children sleepwalk at least once, and 3–4 percent of children have frequent episodes (meaning weekly or monthly). Sleepwalking usually begins when a child is between four and six years of age and peaks between four and eight years. About one-third of children who walk in their sleep will continue to sleepwalk for up to five years; and about 10 percent will continue to sleep walk for ten years.

Approximately 3 percent of children experience sleeps terrors, and they primarily occur during the preschool and elementary school years between the ages of four and twelve years. Sleep terrors are usually more frequent at their initial onset and decrease in rate of recurrence as a child gets older.

Although sleepwalking and sleep terrors can occur at any age, most children outgrow sleep terrors by adolescence because of the normal decrease in slow wave sleep. Although this may be comforting to a parent of an eleven-year-old, it's small consolation if your child is still in preschool.

GROWING OUT OF IT

Most children grow out of sleepwalking and sleep terrors. By age eight, half of all children no longer experience them, and almost all stop having them after puberty, since there is a dramatic decrease in slow wave sleep.

Causes

We don't know exactly what causes sleepwalking or sleep terrors or why children appear to be so confused and frightened during these episodes, although such fascinating phenomena are deserving of more study. But we do know that although they may cause you to have a few more gray hairs, *sleepwalking and sleep terrors are not harmful to children.* Sleep terrors and sleepwalking are truly nothing to worry about, and your main job as a parent is to make sure your child is safe and try to avoid situations that might make an episode more likely to happen.

Sleep terrors and sleepwalking often run in families, so in many cases there is a genetic component. There is an 80–90 percent likelihood that a child with sleepwalking or sleep terrors has a close relative who also has a sleepwalking or sleep terror past. So if your child has sleep terrors, there is a high likelihood that either you or your child's other parent walked in his sleep, talked in his sleep, or had sleep terrors during childhood (or in rare cases still does).

Dan's daughter Lisa had been having sleep terrors every few months since she was three. When Dan finally mentioned it to his mother, she recalled that he had done the same thing for a short time when he was young. His wife also teased him that he still sometimes talked in his sleep, especially when he was very tired.

Triggers

There are certain factors that may increase the likelihood or frequency of sleepwalking or sleep terrors *in a child who is already susceptible to them.* These include:

- **Not getting enough sleep.** Sleep deprivation is the most common trigger for sleepwalking and sleep terrors. When your child is sleep deprived, she is more likely to have the type of sleep (deep sleep) during which these behaviors occur. (One of our former sleep clinic patients, an otherwise mild-mannered and perfectly nice sixteen-year-old boy with a history of sleepwalking, was brought in by his parents after frightening the bejeezus out of them by wandering around the house at night and grabbing knives from the kitchen drawer. He also tore the door off his bedroom closet one night. As it turns out, he was getting only about five hours of sleep since starting a new after-school job and was drinking several six-packs of Mountain Dew a day to keep himself awake. We put him on a strict eight-hour sleep schedule, cut the caffeine, and *voila!* No more middle-of-the night escapades!)

- **An irregular sleep schedule.** Going to bed and getting up at different times every day will also make it more likely that your child will walk in her sleep or have a sleep terror.
- **Frequent night wakings or a late bedtime.** If either of these lead to not getting enough sleep, it's more likely that sleepwalking or a sleep terror will occur.
- **Fever or illness.** For some reason, children are susceptible to parasomnias when they are sick, especially if they have a fever or an ear infection.
- **Some medications.** Some medications may increase the chances that your child will have a sleep terror or sleepwalking episode. Chloral hydrate, a medication that is sometimes prescribed for sleep problems or to sedate children for medical procedures, is one of these. Clonidine, which is also sometimes used as a sleeping pill, is another.
- **Sleeping with a full bladder.** A full bladder can trigger your child to sleepwalk. For some reason, boys are especially susceptible to urinating in inappropriate places when sleepwalking, such as in a closet or out in the backyard. (One of our sleep clinic patients once urinated on his grandfather, who was peacefully sleeping on the living room couch. Talk about a rude awakening!)
- **Sleeping in a different environment.** Sleepwalking and sleep terrors are more likely to occur when your child is sleeping somewhere other than home, such as at a grandparents' house, at a sleepover, or at overnight camp. Be sure to warn grandparents, friends' parents, and camp counselors if your child is susceptible to these behaviors.
- **Sleeping in a noisy environment.** Noise can trigger a parasomnia,

so children who live on noisy streets or in noisy neighborhoods may be more likely to have these behaviors. Household noise can also do it (the kindergartener, mentioned above, was often triggered into a sleep terror episode by the noise of her teenage brother practicing his drums in the next room).

- **Stress.** If your child gets stressed, whether it's because a family pet has died, she's about to start a new school year, or she's just worried about a test, she's likely to get less sleep, which can trigger a parasomnia. It's usually not the stressor itself that leads to the sleepwalking or sleep terror, but rather the sleep deprivation that often accompanies being stressed.
- **Another sleep problem.** If your child has another sleep problem, such as obstructive sleep apnea (see chapter 13), or frequently wakes during the night (see chapter 9), he will be more susceptible to experiencing a parasomnia. Anything that disrupts your child's sleep can trigger a sleep terror or sleepwalking, or may make your child sleep deprived and thus more likely to have one.

Making the Diagnosis

It's important to talk with your child's doctor if your son or daughter seems to be having sleep terrors or sleepwalking episodes. The diagnosis of parasomnias is usually based solely on a parent's report of what happens with their child during the night; it is usually not necessary to do additional testing if the story is classic for sleepwalking or sleep terrors. However, if there is concern about the possibility of another sleep disorder, such as sleep apnea or periodic limb movement disorder (see chapters 13 and 14 for more information), an overnight sleep study may be conducted. There may be times, however, when the description suggests another possible cause for unusual nighttime episodes. If there is any reason to suspect an alternative explanation that would need further evaluation, such as a seizure (this is relatively rare), your doctor may request additional tests, perhaps an EEG ("brain wave"). Because the episodes may occur only infrequently, a homemade videotape of an event that your doctor can then review can be extremely valuable and save a lot of time. It can also be very helpful to keep a diary of your child's sleep for two weeks (a sample sleep diary can be found in appendix A). A sleep diary will help you assess what factors may be triggering the parasomnias, such as sleep deprivation and an irregular sleep schedule.

What Else Could It Be?

Behaviors that occur in the middle of the night have any one of a number of possible explanations, including:

- **Night wakings.** Many children wake up at night and may be upset and agitated if they can't fall back asleep. They may also get out of bed and wander into another room, especially into a parent's room. However, these kids are clearly awake and coherent and know exactly what they are doing.
- **Nightmares.** Nightmares usually occur in the middle of the night or in the early morning hours, when REM sleep is most abundant. In contrast to sleep terrors, a child who is having nightmares often seeks comfort and reassurance from a parent and the next day is able to remember and even describe the bad dream (sometimes in gory detail). She also may have a hard time falling back to sleep after the episode. Nightmares are also a whole lot more common than sleep terrors, so if you're a betting person, the odds are on nightmares. (For more information on nightmares, see chapter 10.)
- **Seizures.** There are rare occasions when it is difficult to differentiate between a nighttime seizure (which are not all that uncommon in children and, despite what you may have heard, are usually quite benign) and a parasomnia. Many children with nighttime seizures have seizures during the day as well, although there are some types of seizures that occur only during sleep. Nighttime seizures often occur as a child is falling asleep or waking up, or in the lighter stages (not deep) of sleep. Most children with seizures do not get out of bed, and the movements during the episode tend to look the same every time. There may be bedwetting directly after the episode. Children with seizures, in contrast to those with parasomnias, are often tired and sleepy the

next day. The bottom line is that your child's doctor will help you determine whether further testing for seizures is necessary.

- **Nighttime anxiety attacks.** Some children wake up during the night with anxiety or "panic" attacks. In most cases, children who have panic attacks are very anxious during the day as well, and many have had some history of trauma. In contrast to children with parasomnias, they generally have quite a vivid memory of the nighttime event.

Sleep Solutions

- **Keep your child safe.** The most important thing that you can do if your child sleepwalks or has sleep terrors is to keep her safe. Make sure that all outside doors are secure. Put up gates at the door of your child's bedroom and at the top of stairs. An alarm can be helpful to make sure that you know your child is up and about and can't leave the house. Any type of alarm will do, from an expensive burglar alarm to a simple bell hung on the door. Ensure that windows, especially second-story or higher, do not open wide enough that your child can jump out of them. And, finally, remove things that are in the way. Clear away anything that your child can step on or trip over.

- **Don't try to awaken your child.** As tempting as it is for parents to try to stop the sleep terror, generally, nothing is gained by trying to awaken your child when she is having one (the same goes for sleepwalking). Although there won't be any permanent damage done if you do manage to wake her up, you may end up making her more agitated and prolonging the episode.

- **Guide your child back to bed.** Try guiding your child gently back to bed while speaking to her in a calm and soothing manner. If she resists, let her be.

- **Try not to interfere too much.** The normal response of parents is to try to comfort their child during one of these episodes. Try to resist doing this. Most children will just get more agitated. It can also make the episode last longer. If your child is about to fall into harm's way, though, be sure to keep your child safe, even if she fights you tooth and nail.

- **Get enough sleep.** Parasomnias are much more likely to happen when your child has not had enough sleep. So increase the amount of sleep that your child is getting and try to not let her become sleep deprived. Moving bedtime to an earlier hour can solve the problem.
- **Keep a regular sleep schedule.** Sleep terrors and sleepwalking are more likely to happen on nights that your child goes to sleep at a time that is different than usual.
- **Don't make it a big deal.** The morning after an episode let your child be your guide in terms of discussing the event. In other words, if she brings it up (chances are she won't remember a thing), reassure her that she is perfectly normal. If not, drop it. Discussing the event is likely to worry her and make her feel embarrassed and self-conscious. She does need to know that she sleepwalks or has sleep terrors, but it shouldn't be the hot topic at the breakfast table (especially with siblings present) the next morning.
- **Consider more aggressive treatment.** In most cases, sleepwalking and sleep terrors require no treatment except for the recommendations given above. In severe cases, however, when there is a possibility that your child may hurt himself or others, when the episodes are very frequent, or when they seriously disrupt your family, additional treatment may be necessary. Treatment may include behavior modification techniques or, rarely, medication. Be sure to speak to your child's doctor if your child has frequent or severe sleep terrors or sleepwalking and you are concerned.

Robert had walked in his sleep off and on since he was four. Now at the age of eight, he was also having sleep terrors. These were scaring his younger brother, who shared a room with him, especially the time that Robert threw a chair across the room. Robert's doctor prescribed a medication (Valium) that helped tremendously. Robert still talks in his sleep once in a while, but everyone in the family sleeps dramatically better.

FACT OR FICTION

It is dangerous to wake a child who is sleepwalking?

Some old wives' tales say that you should never wake a child who is sleepwalking. They never specify why, but it sounds quite ominous. This statement is fiction, in that nothing bad will happen to your child if you wake her when she is sleepwalking or having a sleep terror. On the fact side, though, we do not recommend waking your child, because it will simply agitate your child and make the entire episode last longer. It is much better to let the event run its course, neither speaking to your child nor touching her. You will be surprised how much shorter it will last if you do not intervene. Hard to do as a parent, but worth it.

13

Snoring and Snorting:
Sleep Apnea and Other Breathing Problems During Sleep

"Doctor, you have to help me. Every night Ryan stops breathing. It lasts so long that I think that he won't start breathing again. I have him sleep with me so that I can shake him to make him breathe whenever he stops. He tosses and turns all night and snores so loudly I can hear it in the next room. He can't be getting a good night's sleep and I know I'm not!"

*O*bstructive sleep apnea (OSA) is a sleep-related breathing problem that occurs in both adults and children. It is relatively more common in young children, particularly between the ages of three and seven, but affects children and adolescents of all ages. In some children, as with Ryan, it's pretty clear that something is really wrong. But many children with OSA go undiagnosed because they have more subtle symptoms, or because their parents (and sometimes their doctor) may not be aware that snoring can be a sign of a serious medical condition. "Snoring? Serious? I know my husband snores up a storm every night, and he seems fine!" But is he really? Many adults with OSA also go for years without seeking medical attention, because they think that snoring, at worst, is just a big nuisance for their bed partner. They chalk up their high blood pressure to having put on a few extra pounds in the last five years, and shrug off nodding off at stoplights to a few too many late nights.

But the truth is that sleep apnea in both adults and kids can have serious short-term and long-term consequences. Obstructive sleep apnea is caused by narrowing or a blockage of the upper airway, which typically becomes much worse during the night. Air squeezing through the narrow airway is what causes the snoring (think of trying to blow air through a collapsed straw). If the airway becomes completely blocked, airflow (and therefore breathing) temporarily stops. The good news is that the decrease in oxygen and increase in carbon dioxide in the body caused by lack of breathing are a signal to the brain that breathing has stopped. Fortunately, the brain is then smart enough to signal the body to briefly awaken and restart breathing. This cycle can repeat itself over and over again throughout the night. The bad news is that lack of oxygen, even brief, is not good for anyone, but is particularly bad for the developing brain. And the brief awakenings, as life-saving as they are and even if you are not fully aware of them, repeatedly disrupt sleep and make for some pretty poor sleep quality. Imagine someone poking you in the arm thirty or forty times throughout the night. You would feel exhausted the next day too! So the double-whammy combination of not enough oxygen and too little sleep is what leads to most of the daytime problems (such as sleepiness, irritability, and poor attention) associated with OSA.

A PARENT'S WORST FEAR

A parent's worst fear is that their child will stop breathing when he is asleep and die. Although they sound similar, obstructive sleep apnea is *not* the same kind of apnea that occurs in some premature babies or is associated with SIDS (sudden infant death syndrome). A child (or adult) with OSA will *always* start breathing again after the pause.

The most common reason for breathing problems during sleep in children is related to having large tonsils and adenoids that block the upper airway.

OBSTRUCTIVE SLEEP APNEA

Obstructive sleep apnea (OSA) is a common sleep disorder in children and adolescents that is characterized by frequent breathing pauses, in which your child stops breathing for brief periods. These breathing pauses lead to multiple arousals that disrupt sleep throughout the night. Such arousals cause a poor night's sleep and daytime sleepiness the next day. In children, this breathing problem is usually related to enlarged tonsils and adenoids.

The Many Faces of Sleep-Disordered Breathing

Throughout this chapter we will use the term OSA to refer to nighttime breathing problems in children. It is important, however, to understand that obstructive sleep apnea is at one end of a spectrum of related types of breathing problems during sleep. All of these fall under the catchall phrase "sleep-disordered breathing." The various disorders are described below in order of increasing severity:

- **"Simple" Snoring:** Some children simply snore without any additional breathing problems, like apnea. Until recently it was thought that snoring alone, although annoying, was not a big deal in children. However, recent research is starting to question this assumption. It seems that there may be a link between snoring (with or without associated breathing problems) and poor school performance.

FACT OR FICTION?

Snoring means a child is getting a good night's sleep.

Actually, children (and adults, too) shouldn't snore. And in some cases, snoring may be a sign of a more serious breathing problem, obstructive sleep apnea.

- **Upper airway resistance syndrome (UARS):** *Upper airway resistance syndrome* is the term used when there are mild breathing problems during sleep. UARS has the same basic causes as OSA (namely large tonsils and adenoids) and is treated in the same way. Symptoms of UARS include snoring, some difficulty breathing (you may see or hear your child breathing noisily and his chest moving up and down as he works hard to breathe), and relatively minor changes in the flow of air during sleep. A child with UARS may wake up momentarily after snoring, which will disrupt his sleep and make him sleepy during the day. The main distinction between UARS and OSA is that UARS doesn't show up on a normal sleep study test (see "Making the Diagnosis" on page 159), but instead requires special testing to diagnose.

- **Hypopneas:** The term *hypopneas* is used when there are breathing problems during sleep, but breathing doesn't totally stop ("hypo" meaning "less than" + "apnea," meaning absence of breathing). This is the most common pattern of sleep-disordered breathing in children. Which means that you may be less likely to hear the clear pauses in breathing in kids with OSA than in adults with OSA (what you are more likely to hear in children is snoring interrupted by choking and gasping noises). However, even though they are less severe, repeated hypopneas throughout the night have pretty much the same consequences (decreased oxygen, disrupted sleep) as frequent apneas.
- **Obstructive sleep apnea (OSA):** Obstructive sleep apnea is the full-blown picture. It includes snoring and breathing pauses in which breathing literally stops for a few moments, and your child fully or partially awakens following the stopped breath (usually just for a few seconds). OSA is the sleep-disordered breathing pattern most common in adolescents and adults.

WHAT OBSTRUCTIVE SLEEP APNEA LOOKS LIKE

Child snores. . . .
    Child stops breathing. . . .
        Child briefly wakes up. . . .
            Child moves. . . .
                Child returns to sleep . . . .

Clues

The most common symptoms of obstructive sleep apnea in children and adolescents are loud snoring, breathing pauses, and difficulty in breathing during sleep. Many children who snore do *not* have obstructive sleep apnea (about one in ten do), but very few children with obstructive sleep apnea do *not* snore.

DOES YOUR CHILD HAVE OBSTRUCTIVE SLEEP APNEA?

• While sleeping, does your child:
    ❏ snore more than half the time?
    ❏ snore loudly?
    ❏ have heavy or loud breathing?
    ❏ have trouble breathing, or struggle to breathe?

• Have you ever seen your child stop breathing during the night?

• Does your child:
    ❏ tend to breathe through his/her mouth during the day?
    ❏ Have a dry mouth when s/he wakes up in the morning?
    ❏ Occasionally wet the bed (if over age six)?
    ❏ Have a problem with sleepiness during the day?

• Is it hard to wake your child up in the morning?

If you answered yes to three or more of these questions, be sure to speak with your child's doctor.

Common *nighttime* symptoms of obstructive sleep apnea include:

- **Loud snoring.** Most children with OSA snore loudly and snore every night. However, the volume and frequency of the snoring does not necessarily predict whether or not a particular child has OSA or is just sawing a whole lot of wood. Some children may snore loudly only when they are sleeping on their backs. Other children snore only when they have a cold or allergies.
- **Breathing pauses.** You may literally see your child stop breathing when she sleeps. Other indications of breathing pauses are choking, gasping, and snorting during the night.

HOW WORRIED ARE YOU ABOUT YOUR CHILD'S BREATHING?

Interestingly, it seems that the best predictor of severe sleep apnea is how worried a parent is at night. If you often stay with your child when he sleeps so that you can watch over him all night and shake him if he stops breathing, this is a fairly good indicator that your child has severe obstructive sleep apnea

- **Struggling to breathe.** You may notice that your child has a difficult time breathing or is struggling to breathe when she is asleep. Rather than see her chest and abdomen moving together when she breathes, you may even see them moving in opposite directions.
- **Restless sleep.** Your child may be a restless sleeper, moving about frequently throughout the night. This restlessness occurs because your child is likely to move and shift position every time she briefly wakes up following a breathing pause.
- **Sweating.** Your child may sweat when she sleeps. Some believe that children with sleep apnea are more likely to sweat when they sleep because they are working so hard to breathe.
- **Odd sleeping position.** Your child may sleep sitting up, sleep propped up with lots of pillows, or even sleep with her head hanging off the side of the bed. These are all ways that your child is trying keep her airway open so that she can breathe easier.

That's the fairly obvious part in recognizing possible OSA in kids. What is often not at all obvious, unless you know what to look for and why, are some of the following daytime *symptoms* of OSA:

- **Mouth breathing.** Your child may breathe through her mouth during the day, which is often an indication that large adenoids are blocking the air coming in through the nose. If your child's adenoids are big or she has allergies with nasal congestion, she may not be able to breathe well through her nose, so she keeps her mouth open.
- **Dry mouth.** Your child may also complain of having a dry mouth and frequently needs a drink during the day and during the night.
- **Morning headaches.** Some children report headaches in the morning. This is related to the breathing problems at night. The headache will likely go away within an hour or two.
- **Chronic stuffy nose.** Your child may often have a stuffy nose, which can contribute to breathing problems at night.
- **Frequent infections.** Many children with OSA also have frequent ear infections and sinusitis.

- **Nasal speech.** You may notice that your child often has a nasal voice, again because of large adenoids. To check if your child's voice is nasal, ask him to say the following words normally and then while pinching his nose closed: "ninety-nine," "Mickey Mouse," and "my name is money." You should hear a difference. If you don't, it can be an indication of blocked nasal passages.
- **Difficulty swallowing.** Some children with OSA also have trouble swallowing and eating. This can be related to large tonsils that get in the way when your child is eating. Your child may also have a poor appetite.
- **Daytime sleepiness.** Your child may be sleepy during the day, as a result of her sleep being disrupted throughout the night. Some classic signs of sleepiness are difficulty waking up in the morning or falling asleep at school or other times throughout the day.
- **Naps.** Younger children with sleep apnea may take longer naps than other children their age or still be napping after you would expect them to no longer be napping. Children with sleep apnea may also take unplanned naps, such as falling asleep while watching television or doing homework. They may fall asleep in the car.
- **Behavior problems.** Rather than appearing sleepy, children's sleepiness may reveal itself as behavior problems or other problems during the day. These behaviors may include mood changes, such as being irritable, cranky, impatient, having mood swings, being moody, or even being depressed or anxious. Your child may also have problems paying attention and be easily distracted. She may be impulsive. Aggression and being overactive are common, with some children even having behaviors during the day that look like attention-deficit/hyperactivity disorder (ADHD; see chapter 17 for more information on the connection between sleep and ADHD). Academic problems as a result of these behavioral issues are also common.

OSA SYMPTOMS TO LOOK FOR IN YOUR CHILD

- Snoring
- Breathing pauses during sleep or difficulty breathing during sleep
- Mouth breathing
- Noisy breathing
- Restless sleep
- Sweating during sleep
- Morning headaches
- Difficulty waking in the morning
- Daytime sleepiness
- Daytime behavior problems, especially overactivity and irritability
- Academic problems
- Nasal voice

Other Possible Problems

Children with sleep apnea may also have other problems.

- **Bedwetting.** Some children with sleep apnea have a difficult time staying dry at night. In fact, OSA should be suspected as the culprit if your child who for years has been toilet trained at night starts wetting the bed again. Once the sleep apnea is treated, many children become dry at night as a result.
- **Growth issues.** Some children with OSA are small for their age. These growth problems may be caused by a combination of things, including a poor appetite, increased metabolism from working so hard to breathe during the night, and interruption of the normal release of growth hormone that occurs during sleep. Alternatively, more and more of the children we are seeing for obstructive sleep apnea are overweight and even obese.
- **Parasomnias.** Sleepwalking and sleep terrors are more common in children with OSA. An episode can be triggered by a pause in breathing or can be the result of the sleep deprivation that often goes

along with OSA. (For more information on these sleep problems, see chapter 12.)

- **Bedtime problems and night wakings.** Bedtime problems and night wakings occur in about 25 percent of children with OSA. Night wakings, especially, may be related to obstructive sleep apnea, in that a child who has apnea is more likely to wake up at night. However, a child who wakes up because of a breathing issue should be able to return to sleep on his own, so there is often an added behavioral issue. (See chapters 8 and 9 on bedtime problems and night wakings.)

Seven-year-old Kirk had always snored loudly and sometimes seemed to have problems breathing at night. He still insisted that one of his parents stay with him at bedtime until he was asleep. Two or three times a night, he would come into their bedroom and need one of them to come stay with him until he fell back to sleep. After treating his sleep apnea, he still woke up at least once a night and woke his parents up to stay with him.

How Common Is It?

Studies have shown that about 20 percent of children occasionally snore at night, while 10 percent snore almost every single night. Obstructive sleep apnea occurs in about 1 to 3 percent of preschoolers. Unfortunately there is little data on how common OSA is in other age groups, although at least 50 percent of the children we evaluate in our sleep clinic for OSA are school-aged and somewhere around 10 percent are teenagers, and these numbers appear to be growing.

Causes

In most children, sleep apnea is caused by large tonsils or adenoids, which can block the airway. The reason obstructive sleep apnea is most common in children between the ages of three and six is because of the combination of normally large tonsils and a small airway. As children get older, their tonsils naturally start to shrink and their airway gets larger.

SIZE DOESN'T COUNT AFTER ALL

A number of studies have shown that there is not always a direct relationship between the size of a child's tonsils and adenoids and whether or not he has obstructive sleep apnea. Children with very large tonsils and adenoids may not always have obstructive sleep apnea, and children with small tonsils and adenoids may.

There are also some additional "risk factors" that may raise or lower the odds your child will have obstructive sleep apnea:

- **Age.** Breathing problems during sleep can occur at any age, but those that are related to big tonsils and adenoids are most likely between two and seven years of age, when the tonsils and adenoids are typically at their largest. OSA related to weight issues is more likely to occur during adolescence, when sleep apnea is more like "adult" obstructive sleep apnea.
- **Gender.** Although obstructive sleep apnea occurs equally in boys and girls before puberty, boys seem to be more likely to have sleep apnea after puberty (much like the pattern in adult men and women).
- **Ethnicity.** Some research suggests that African-American children may be at a higher risk for developing sleep apnea.
- **Family history.** It's common for children with sleep apnea to have another family member who also snores loudly or has sleep apnea (whether or not it has been diagnosed by a doctor).
- **Weight issues.** The best predictor of whether or not an adult man is likely to have OSA is a collar size of seventeen inches and above. Obesity is far and away the most common risk factor for OSA in adults. As the epidemic of childhood obesity in the United States grows, we are seeing more and more children who have sleep-disordered breathing problems related to their weight. And it's not only obese kids; it's kids who are simply overweight as well. And being even moderately overweight, in a child who already has large tonsils and adenoids, may "tip the scales" if you will, toward OSA.

- **Allergies and asthma.** Children with seasonal and environmental allergies, asthma, or frequent sinus infections may also be at increased risk for obstructive sleep apnea.
- **Sickle cell disease.** There is some evidence to suggest that children with sickle cell disease may have a higher risk of OSA. In addition, OSA may be more dangerous in these children, because the associated decrease in oxygen can trigger a "sickle crisis."
- **Other medical conditions.** Certain medical problems, many of which are present at birth, make it more likely that a particular child will have OSA. Children who are at high risk for sleep apnea include those with a particularly narrow face (and thus narrow airway) and children with cleft palate. Because of their facial structure and low muscle tone, children with Down syndrome are particularly susceptible to developing OSA (up to 70 percent, by some estimates), as are children with achondroplasia (dwarfism). Any condition with low muscle tone (such as muscular dystrophy, congenital hypotonias) has a higher than normal risk of OSA. Although rare in children, hypothyroidism (low thyroid hormone) increases the risk of OSA. In addition, gastroesophageal reflux, because it can irritate the back of the throat and upper airway and cause some swelling, may also contribute to OSA.

THE OBESITY EPIDEMIC AND SLEEP APNEA

We all know that more and more children these days are overweight or obese. Since being overweight increases the risk of sleep apnea, the prevalence of sleep apnea in children is also increasing.

Making the Diagnosis

Most children with symptoms of obstructive sleep apnea require an overnight sleep study to confirm the diagnosis. An overnight sleep study, which is done in a specialized sleep laboratory, monitors breathing, heart rate, and sleep throughout the night.

WHY DOES MY CHILD NEED A SLEEP STUDY?

Although your child's symptoms are important in making the diagnosis of obstructive sleep apnea, there is still no way to know for sure whether or not your child has sleep apnea or is just snoring. An overnight sleep study is the only way to know for sure. An overnight sleep study also gives us important information about how severe the OSA is, which might affect treatment options.

There are some differing opinions about whether or not a sleep study is absolutely necessary before taking out the tonsils and adenoids in a child with OSA. Because symptoms alone do not accurately predict which snoring child has OSA and which child does not, the American Academy of Pediatrics has recommended that all children who habitually snore have an overnight sleep study done as part of the evaluation for OSA. However, there are some physicians who feel that a sleep study is not always necessary in very clear-cut cases. And if your child has frequent strep throat or there are other reasons for removing your child's tonsils and adenoids, then a sleep study may not always be necessary. Until we have more studies to sort this out, your best bet is to talk to your doctor about the benefits and drawbacks of having your child undergo a sleep study.

A physical exam by your child's doctor is also important to help understand what may be contributing to your child's breathing problems. Allergies, asthma, frequent tonsillitis, and sinus infections can all be causes and treated. Your child's doctor will also be able to get a sense of the size of your child's tonsils (special equipment is required to see the adenoids, and this is usually only done by an ear, nose, and throat specialist). Your child's doctor may also request a lateral neck X-ray to determine whether or not your child's adenoids are large. This X-ray can also help determine the size of your child's airway and tongue. All of these can be important in determining whether your child has sleep apnea and what the best treatment will be.

OVERNIGHT SLEEP STUDY

An overnight sleep study is formally called a *polysomnogram* (PSG). Most sleep studies are done in a specialized lab at a hospital or sleep center, although sometimes they are conducted at home. For the sleep study, you will be asked to arrive with your child two or three hours before his normal bedtime. A technician will glue or tape to your child's skin a number of sensors and monitors. These will measure your child's heart rate, breathing rate, leg movements, eye movements, and brain waves. Nothing that is put on your child will hurt, although sometimes it takes children or adolescents a little while to get used to all the stuff stuck on them (be sure to bring your camera!). All of these measurements will help evaluate when your child falls asleep, the stages of sleep, and whether or not your child has a sleep disorder. Your child will be monitored all night by a technician, and an infrared camera will record your child's sleep. In most centers, a parent will need to stay, too, and there is often a cot in the room for you to get some sleep (although a warning—if you snore, you may be asked to wait somewhere else; they want to hear whether your child snores, not you!).

Sometimes a second test will be done the next day, called a *multiple sleep latency test* (MSLT). This test will evaluate whether your child or adolescent is sleepy during the day. An MSLT usually consists of four or five twenty-minute naps at two-hour intervals. So, if your child wakes up at 7:00 AM, the naps will occur at 9:00, 11:00, 1:00, 3:00, and possibly 5:00. Your child will be asked to lie down, shut his eyes, and try to fall asleep. The length of time it takes your child to fall asleep will be measured. If your child falls asleep, he will be woken up after fifteen or twenty minutes. If he doesn't fall asleep, he'll be asked to get out of bed after twenty minutes.

It usually takes about a week for the results from the sleep study and/or MSLT to be compiled.

OVERNIGHT SLEEP STUDY TERMS

If your child undergoes an overnight sleep study, it can be helpful to understand the terms that are most commonly used:

Apnea/hypopnea index: This index is the number of apnea and hypopnea events per hour of sleep and is often referred to as AHI. An apnea is when your child totally stops breathing, and a *hypopnea* is when your child partially stops breathing. A report will typically say "AHI = 4.6." This means that averaged across the night, your child had 4.6 apnea and hypopnea events per hour. There is no absolute universal standard in children, but we usually say that an AHI that is greater than 5 in any age child indicates definite OSA, and an AHI between 1 and 5 in younger children indicates possible OSA.

Apnea index (AI): An apnea index is the average number of apnea events (breathing pauses) per hour. The total number of apnea events is divided by the number of hours of sleep to give an average. An apnea index of over 1.0 per hour is usually considered a problem.

Arousal index: This is an average of the number of times your child had an arousal (briefly woke up) per hour throughout the night. An arousal is defined as any time that that your child wakes up for three or more seconds. Watching your child, you probably wouldn't even notice these brief arousals. A standard arousal index that is considered high is over fifteen per hour in children. A high arousal index can be an indication of a breathing problem that is waking your child. Some children have a high arousal index during a sleep study just from being uncomfortable.

Oxygen saturation: These numbers indicate your child's baseline oxygen level (normal is around 95–100 percent), and how low and how frequently it dips during the night.

Carbon dioxide: Many sleep labs also measure the level of carbon dioxide in the blood or in the lungs, which if high, can be another indication that there is a breathing problem

What Else Could It Be?

- **Difficulty breathing during sleep** can be caused by many other medical problems, such as allergies, asthma, and reflux.

- **Daytime sleepiness** can also be caused by many other things. The number one cause of sleepiness is not getting enough sleep (obvious, but true). Other sleep disorders can also cause sleepiness during the day, such as narcolepsy (see chapter 16) and periodic limb movement disorder (see chapter 14). Being sleepy or tired during the day can also be related to emotional issues, such as depression and anxiety (see chapter 19), as well as medical problems (see chapter 19).

Sleep Solutions

There are many different potential treatments for snoring and sleep apnea. Discuss with your doctor all the different treatment options and which one(s) will be best for your child.

- **Remove the tonsils and adenoids.** For most children with sleep apnea, removing the tonsils and adenoids, if they are enlarged, takes care of the problem. You will be sent to an ear, nose, and throat specialist, who will evaluate your child for surgery. Research shows that surgery to remove the tonsils and adenoids resolves sleep apnea in 70 to 90 percent of children. Removing both the tonsils and adenoids is usually recommended to avoid any future symptoms. Be forewarned, though, that the adenoids can grow back after surgery.

   If your child has severe sleep apnea, or other medical problems, the doctors may decide to keep your child in the hospital overnight after the surgery. This will allow them to closely monitor your child for any breathing problems related to swelling from the surgery. Also, your child's symptoms may take six to eight weeks to completely go away, since there is often some swelling after the surgery.

Madeline had been snoring since she was two years old. Her snoring was much worse now and her second-grade teacher recently commented that Madeline was having problems concentrating in school and getting her work done. Her parents took her to a sleep specialist to check for sleep apnea. An overnight sleep study found that Madeline had an apnea index of 9.2. That is, she stopped breathing more than nine times an hour. Surgery was scheduled over spring break. It made a world of difference. Madeline was now more easily awakened to get up for school in the morning, her appetite increased, and her teacher noticed a dramatic improvement in her behavior during the day. She was getting her schoolwork done, and she was less likely to get frustrated with her friends.

- **Other surgical procedures.** There are other surgical procedures that your doctor may suggest, such as if your child has a deviated septum or other problems.
- **Use continuous positive airway pressure** (CPAP). Nasal CPAP is the most common treatment for obstructive sleep apnea in adults. CPAP involves wearing a mask over the nose and/or mouth during sleep that is hooked up by tubing to a machine that keeps the airway open by blowing air under pressure into the mask (think of it as a kind of "backwards vacuum cleaner"). CPAP can be used successfully with children and adolescents, even children as young as a year old. CPAP may be recommended if removing the adenoids and tonsils is not indicated (if your child's tonsils and adenoids are very small or have already been removed), if surgery was not completely effective, if your child is obese, or if your child has other medical issues. Getting your child to wear the CPAP mask is the key to its success. But even children with significant developmental delays or Down syndrome can be successful CPAP users. Your doctor can help you come up with a plan to get your child used to the mask and to keeping it on all night.

Ricky, a seven-year-old with Down syndrome, had severe sleep apnea. His doctor recommended that he wear a CPAP mask at night to help him breathe. The first night they tried it in the lab was a total disaster. Ricky screamed and had a temper tantrum. His parents finally gave up after several hours and just went home. They then spent the next few weeks getting Ricky used to the mask. At first they put it on one of his favorite stuffed animals and had the teddy bear sleep with him at night. They then started having Ricky wear just the mask by itself whenever he watched a favorite video. Every time Ricky took off the mask, they turned off the video. Soon, Ricky was wearing it for longer and longer periods. Once he was comfortable with the mask, they tried again at night. This time went much more smoothly, and Ricky now earns stickers for wearing his "breathing mask" all night.

- **Get fit and trim.** If your child is overweight, it's important to help him lose weight. Talk with his doctor or a nutritionist about healthy eating habits and an exercise program for your child. Decrease junk foods and desserts, take family bike rides or an evening walk, get rid of soda and fruit juices, have healthy snacks around the house, such as yummy fruits and vegetables, and avoid fast-food restaurants. Not only will these changes help your child, but they also will benefit everyone in the family.
- **Get him off his back.** Some children and adolescents snore or have breathing problems only if they sleep on their back. If this is the case with your child, you can try sewing a tennis ball into a pocket on his pajama top or T-shirt that should then be worn backward to bed. This will prevent your child from sleeping on his back.
- **Treat the allergies.** Your doctor may recommend or prescribe a medication such as a nasal spray if your child is often congested. Allergy medications can also be very helpful. However, except in very mild cases, these medications will not completely solve the problem. Because both asthma and reflux can make OSA worse, these conditions, if present, should be aggressively treated.
- **Stay out of trouble.** On the other hand, your child should avoid anything that is sedating, such as Benadryl or alcohol, as they can make your child's sleep apnea worse. Your child should also not be exposed to cigarette smoke, which can make it more difficult for him to breathe.
- **See a dentist.** Although generally not used in children, sometimes a dental appliance may be recommended for treating OSA. Some appliances move your child's lower jaw forward, helping him to

breathe. An orthodontist or dentist typically fits children and adolescents for these devices.

- **Treat other sleep problems.** Many children with breathing problems at night also have other sleep problems, such as frequently waking up during the night or refusing to go to bed. It's important that you also resolve these problems to help your child get the best night's sleep possible.

- **Be a good role model.** Since OSA tends to run in families, common sense would tell us that the odds of a child with OSA having a parent with OSA are pretty high. We see many parents who bring their child in for an evaluation and just "happen to mention" that they snore as well (this is typically the mom who reports that her husband keeps her awake all night with his snoring) and "might" have dozed off at the wheel a time or two. But they are usually quick to add, "It's no big deal." It is a big deal. You could be risking high blood pressure, even a heart attack, a stroke, or a car accident by not getting this checked out. Get seen and get treated!

Making the Decision Whether to Treat

The decision of whether and how to treat snoring or obstructive sleep apnea depends on both the severity and the cause. There are different measures of severity. It can include the degree of your child's symptoms, the results of the sleep study, and the degree to which snoring or sleep apnea is affecting your child's life. A child who barely snores, seems to have few problems breathing, has no problems during the day, but has an apnea index of 3.1 may not warrant treatment. On the other hand, it may be worth treating a child who snores loudly, seems to struggle to breathe, has huge tonsils, and has problems paying attention in school but only has an apnea index of 1.6.

Benjamin was such a loud snorer that it was a family joke. However, a sleep study showed that he didn't have sleep apnea and was getting a good night's sleep despite his snoring. It was recommended that they do nothing about his snoring.

One day after a sleepover, Sophia's aunt commented that Sophia seemed to be quite restless at night and that she sometimes seemed to have problems breathing. Although her mother had never noticed, she took Sophia to the doctor. After an X-ray showed that Sophia had huge adenoids, her doctor scheduled a sleep study. The sleep study showed that Sophia had severe sleep apnea, and surgery was recommended. Even though her mother barely noticed a difference in Sophia's sleep at night, she saw a huge improvement in Sophia's behavior during the day. Sophia was no longer cranky, and she stopped complaining that she was always "too tired" to do anything.

Long-Term

Studies find that for most children, obstructive sleep apnea completely resolves after treatment and there are no further problems. At the same time, these studies show that children whose sleep apnea is left untreated or only partially treated often continue to have daytime symptoms and problems with learning and behavior. In one study, children who were treated for their OSA and had previously been in the bottom 10 percent of their elementary school class gained a half-grade in academic performance after treatment. The kids who were not treated stayed put. It is hoped that future studies will provide more information about which children are likely to benefit from treatment and which treatments work best.

WHO SNORES THE LOUDEST IN YOUR FAMILY?

If anyone else in your family snores loudly or has problems breathing while asleep, be sure to have that person checked for sleep apnea too. Many times, the mother or the father of a child with sleep apnea has the same problem. It's just as important for adults to get treated for sleep apnea.

14

Jumping and Jiving:
Restless Legs Syndrome and Periodic Limb
Movement Disorder

Leanna's mother and her grandfather have both been diagnosed with restless legs syndrome. Her mother is now concerned that nine-year-old Leanna's difficulties in falling asleep at night may be for the same reason.

Eric is twelve years old. He falls asleep with no problem at 9:00, but is difficult to awaken at 7:15 on school days. Eric is a very restless sleeper, and both his twin brother and his parents refuse to share a bed with him on family vacations because he is all over the bed and kicks them all night.

*R*estless legs syndrome, often referred to as RLS, is a sleep-related movement disorder that occurs in both adults and children. The child or adolescent with RLS experiences uncomfortable sensations in his legs when sitting still or resting. These sensations are usually described as creepy, crawly, tingling, "pins and needles-like" or, less commonly, painful. Some parents interpret their child's complaints as "growing pains." To relieve the discomfort, children or adolescents with restless legs syndrome usually have an overwhelming urge to move their legs, whether stretching them, getting up and walking or running around, or simply tossing and turning. In addition, they may rub their legs or ask someone else to do it to make them feel better. Because of the discomfort and frequent leg movements, it often takes a long time for children and adolescents with restless legs syndrome to fall asleep at bedtime. Ironically, the precise things you need to do in order to fall asleep (relax, stay still, rest) are the very same things that are most likely to cause the RLS symptoms. Conversely, activity and moving are the two things that relieve the uncomfortable leg sensations, but they also make it nearly impossible to fall asleep. Unfortunately, parents (understandably) may interpret such activity and movement as bedtime resistance or as difficulty in falling asleep for other reasons. During the day, many parents also complain that their child can't sit still, or that he is always moving or fidgeting.

It seemed impossible to get five-year-old Michael settled down at bedtime. He was always getting in and out of his bed once the lights were turned off. His parents referred to him as the "jumping bean." At a recent doctor's visit, after his doctor asked him if anything ever hurt, he said that his legs felt "yucky" at bedtime. His parents were stunned, as he had never mentioned this to them.

RESTLESS LEGS SYNDROME

Restless legs syndrome is characterized by uncomfortable sensations in the legs, resulting in movement to relieve the feeling. The discomfort is usually worse or only present at night, especially at bedtime.

A second sleep disorder that often goes along with restless legs syndrome is called *periodic limb movement disorder* (PLMD). This is also a movement disorder, but it is one that occurs when a child is sleeping rather than when he is trying to fall asleep. The movements are described as leg kicks or twitches during sleep, and they tend to occur in spurts of at least several kicks or twitches in a row, at intervals of about every twenty to forty seconds. These clusters of movements can last from a few minutes to a few hours. Unlike restless legs syndrome, a child with PLMD is usually not aware of the symptoms or the movements, although a parent may observe kicking and restless sleep. The movements may appear as brief muscle twitches, jerking movements, or simply an upward flexing of the feet. Periodic limb movement disorder can result in frequent brief awakenings or arousals throughout the night, disrupting sleep and leading to daytime sleepiness. Sometimes the complaint that brings the child with PLMD in to see a doctor is daytime fatigue or mood or attention problems resulting from the child's disturbed sleep, rather than the sleep symptoms themselves.

PERIODIC LIMB MOVEMENT DISORDER

Periodic limb movement disorder is characterized by periods during the night of repetitive limb movements (usually in the legs, but can also occur in the arms). These movements may briefly wake your child.

Sondra couldn't understand why her nine-year-old son, Andrew, always seemed tired during the day. He went to bed at 8:30 and fell asleep quickly. However, she still had a hard time waking him in the morning at 7:30 for school. It was a family joke that Andrew was more active asleep than awake. He always seemed to be moving around, and everyone refused to share a bed with him, since they frequently got kicked.

Restless legs syndrome and periodic limb movement disorder often occur together. Studies in adults indicate that 70 to 90 percent of adults with restless legs syndrome have periodic limb movement disorder. In contrast, only 20 to 30 percent of people with periodic limb movement disorder also have restless legs syndrome. Comparable studies have not been conducted with children or adolescents, but it is expected that the relationship between these two sleep disorders is similar.

It's important to note that these two disorders have only recently been recognized in children and adolescents. Both disorders are probably much more common in children and adolescents than was previously thought. Therefore, if your child has problems falling asleep, wakes at night, is a restless sleeper, or is frequently sleepy during the day for no identifiable reason, the possibility of restless legs syndrome or periodic limb movement disorder should be considered.

How Common Is It?

Surprisingly, restless legs syndrome and periodic limb movement disorder are quite common in adults. In adults, restless legs syndrome is estimated to occur in about 5 to 15 percent of the general population. The percentage of adults who have PLMD increases with age (5 percent of adults ages 30 to 50, 29 percent in adults 50 to 64, and 44 percent in those over 65). The prevalence of restless legs syndrome and of periodic limb movement disorder in the pediatric population is unknown, although one recent study found that of more than eight hundred children surveyed 17 percent reported "restless legs at night." Furthermore, about 40 percent of adults with restless legs syndrome report the onset of symptoms before age twenty, so there is every reason to think these disorders are quite common in children and teens as well.

Common, yes. But commonly *diagnosed,* no. Despite the fact that one in every ten adults has RLS, many people have symptoms for years before they are diagnosed. Some are never diagnosed at all. There's a bit of a conspiracy of silence to account for this. Patients don't think their symptoms are related to a medical condition or are embarrassed by them and so don't bring them to the attention of their doctor. Doctors often know very little about these disorders and rarely ask about potential symptoms (unfortunately, this same situation exists with many of the sleep disorders discussed in this book). RLS is even less likely to be diagnosed in children, because many physicians and parents are simply unaware that this condition even exists in kids.

Several studies have also found that periodic limb movements occur in nearly a quarter of children who are diagnosed with ADHD. Other recent studies have found an association between hyperactivity and periodic limb movements. It is not currently known whether RLS and PLMD actually cause the ADHD symptoms or if ADHD and RLS/PLMD just tend to occur in the same people. The percentage of children with ADHD who also have RLS and PLMD is still not known (see chapter 17 for more information).

Causes

The cause of restless legs syndrome and periodic limb movement disorder is not completely understood, although both are thought to be related to a decrease in the level of a body chemical called *dopamine.* RLS can run in families, and thus in these cases it's probably genetic. Most adults with restless legs syndrome have a family member with the same disorder, and the risk of developing RLS is six to seven times higher in close relatives of those with RLS.

RLS and PLMD can be related to anemia, caused by a low level of iron or folic acid. Some children with chronic diseases, such as diabetes and kidney disease, are at risk for developing RLS. Additionally, children with leukemia are at increased risk for PLMD. Pregnancy is another condition in which RLS and PLMD are more frequent, and pregnancy can make existing RLS or PLMD worse. About 15–25 percent of pregnant women develop RLS symptoms.

Finally, there are some factors that can exacerbate both problems. Caffeine, alcohol, and certain medications can all make RLS and PLMD worse. Obstructive sleep apnea (see chapter 13) can also trigger periodic limb movements during sleep.

Clues

The symptoms of *restless legs syndrome* may include any and all of the following:

- **Leg discomfort.** Your child may describe uncomfortable feelings in his legs. Some children use words such as "creepy," "crawly," "painful," or "tingling" to describe these feelings. These feelings usually occur at bedtime but can also be present at other times when sitting still, such as during long car or airplane rides or when watching a movie.
- **Leg movements.** To relieve the uncomfortable sensations in his legs, your child may have an irresistible urge to move his legs, whether it is tossing and turning while lying in bed or walking or running about at bedtime. Rarely are these leg sensations described as "painful," although younger children may not be able to accurately explain the feelings in their legs. Your child may also state that these feelings are "inside" or deep within his legs.
- **Sleep disruption.** Your child may take a long time to fall asleep because of the leg discomfort and need to move. He may also have difficulty staying asleep.
- **Bedtime behavior problems.** Because the RLS symptoms peak at bedtime and children have difficulty settling and falling asleep, some children are considered a problem at bedtime.
- **Daytime sleepiness.** The difficulties falling asleep and staying asleep can result in significant daytime sleepiness related to getting inadequate or poor quality sleep.

- **Behavior and academic problems.** In some children, daytime sleepiness gets played out as behavior problems, such as being hyperactive, impulsive, or irritable, as well as difficulties in school.

WORDS KIDS USE TO DESCRIBE RESTLESS LEGS SYNDROME

Creepy	Gotta moves	Itchy bones
Crawly	Heebie-Jeebies	Crazy legs
Pulling	Electric current	Like iced tea
Jumpies		

- **Difficulty sitting still.** Your child may have symptoms during the day, too, making it difficult for him to sit still. This can occur during long car rides, plane flights, movies, or even when having to sit still in school. Your child may be constantly jiggling or moving his legs.

Although many children and adolescents with *periodic limb movement disorder* do not report any symptoms, because they are asleep and are thus unaware of them, symptoms may include any of the following:

- **Leg movements.** Although your child or adolescent will probably not be aware of these movements, repetitive leg movements in sleep characterize periodic limb movement disorder.
- **Sleep disruption.** Your child may wake up at night, as a result of being awakened from the leg kicks.
- **Restless sleep.** Your child may be a restless sleeper due to the leg movements and the frequent arousals. Your child's bedcovers may be highly disheveled during the night and in the morning.
- **Daytime sleepiness.** The frequent arousals in sleep can result in significant daytime sleepiness. It may be difficult to wake your child in the morning, or he may complain that he is still tired, even after it seems like he got enough sleep the night before.
- **Behavior and academic problems.** Your child may have daytime

behavior and academic problems, such as hyperactivity, impulsivity, and irritability, which are the result of the disrupted sleep.

COMMON SYMPTOMS OF RESTLESS LEGS SYNDROME AND PERIODIC LIMB MOVEMENT DISORDER

At bedtime
Difficulty falling asleep
Leg movements
Walking, pacing, or running about at bedtime
Bedtime behavior problems
Leg pain
Leg discomfort

During the night
Leg movements
Restless sleep
Nighttime awakenings

Daytime sleepiness
Difficulty waking in the morning
Morning grogginess
Falling asleep in school or at inappropriate times
Need to nap
Mood changes: irritability, low frustration tolerance, impatience, mood swings, depression/anxiety, and social withdrawal
Acting-out behaviors: aggression, hyperactivity
Oppositional and noncompliant behavior
Inattention, poor concentration, distractibility
ADHD-type symptoms
Academic problems

During the day
Leg movements when sitting still or lying down
Inability to sit still for long periods
Leg discomfort

Making the Diagnosis

There is no definitive test for restless legs syndrome, so a diagnosis is made based on the description of symptoms. A screening questionnaire can be found on page 177. To evaluate for RLS, your child's doctor will take a medical history and do a physical examination to exclude other problems. Finally, an overnight sleep study may be recommended to test for other sleep disorders, especially periodic limb movement disorder, since these two disorders often go hand in hand. Blood work may be ordered to check for iron deficiency anemia with a specific test called a *ferritin level*.

Periodic limb movement disorder is diagnosed by overnight sleep study. This will require your child or adolescent to stay overnight in a sleep laboratory. In addition, a medical history and physical examination will be conducted. As with RLS, your doctor may want to check for anemia.

What Else Could It Be?

- **"Growing pains."** No one really knows what growing pains are, but it seems that some children have pain in their legs at various times while they are growing. Some of these children and adolescents may actually have restless legs syndrome.
- **Another sleep disorder.** Taking a long time to fall asleep at night and waking up at night may result from insomnia, bedtime refusal, or general noncompliance (see chapters 8 and 11 for more information on these sleep problems).
- **Daytime sleepiness.** Daytime sleepiness can be caused by other sleep disorders, including obstructive sleep apnea, narcolepsy, and simply not getting enough sleep.
- **Uncomfortable leg sensations.** Your child's leg discomfort may be related to many other conditions, including leg cramps, sore muscles, orthopedic problems, or chronic pain from another medical condition, such as arthritis.
- **Sleep-related movements/restlessness.** Seizures and waking up frequently from sleep apnea (see chapter 13) can also cause children to move during sleep.

SCREENING QUESTIONNAIRE FOR RESTLESS LEGS SYNDROME (RLS)

	YES	NO
Does your child . . .		
Have "growing pains"?	❑	❑
Complain of uncomfortable or funny feelings (creeping, crawling, tingling) in his/her legs?	❑	❑
Notice funny feelings in his/her legs (or they seem worse) when lying down or sitting?	❑	❑
Have partial relief with movement (wiggling feet, toes, or walking)?	❑	❑
Complain that the feelings are worse at night?	❑	❑
Have a lot of fidgeting or wiggling of the feet or toes when sitting or lying down?	❑	❑
Have repeated jerking movements in toes or legs or the whole body while sleeping?	❑	❑
Appear restless while sleeping (thrashing around, banging feet against wall. twisting covers, or falling out of bed)?	❑	❑
Seem more restless, fidgety or hyperactive than most children his/her age?	❑	❑

If you answered "yes" to three or more of these questions, be sure to speak with your child's doctor.

Sleep Solutions

There are a number of things that can help to relieve the symptoms of restless legs syndrome and/or periodic limb movement disorder.

- **Get enough sleep.** It is recommended that children with restless legs syndrome maintain consistent bedtimes and bedtime routines, as well as get adequate nighttime sleep. Fatigue and drowsiness tend to make the symptoms of restless legs syndrome worse.
- **Change bedtime habits.** Given that the leg discomfort gets worse the longer your child lies in bed, it is usually better for her to wait to get into bed until she is ready to turn out the lights and fall asleep. Thus, reading bedtime stories and engaging in other quiet activities should occur in other places, such as in a nearby chair.
- **Reduce the discomfort.** Massage, cold compresses, or a heating pad may give your child temporary relief of the uncomfortable sensations of restless legs syndrome. Walking and stretching can also help.
- **Avoid caffeine.** Caffeine can make restless legs syndrome and periodic limb movement disorder symptoms worse; so all caffeine should be avoided. Caffeine can be found in many sodas and in tea and coffee, but it is also present in chocolate and in some medications (such as Midol and Excedrin). A complete table on the caffeine content of different foods and medications can be found on page 51.
- **Treat anemia.** Low levels of iron or folic acid can contribute to both of these disorders, so your child's doctor may prescribe an iron or folic acid supplement.
- **Try exercise and other techniques.** Moderate exercise up to a few hours before bedtime may suppress symptoms. Biofeedback and relaxation techniques may partially alleviate symptoms and reduce stress. Keeping mentally occupied, especially during long periods of inactivity, should also be encouraged.
- **Avoid triggers.** Caffeine, alcohol, antihistamines, and cold/sinus preparations are known to exacerbate symptoms of restless legs syndrome.

• **Consider medication.** Medication may be recommended for children and adolescents with severe restless legs syndrome and/or periodic limb movement disorder for whom alternative treatments have not been completely successful. A number of different types of medications that can help, including those that increase the level of dopamine, pain relievers, and certain sleep medications. Your child's doctor will help select the medication that is most appropriate.

CRYSTAL BALL

No long-term studies have been conducted on the course of restless legs syndrome or periodic limb movement disorder in children or adolescents. It is likely, however, that restless legs syndrome and periodic limb movement disorder are chronic, lifelong disorders, although children and adolescents with minimum symptoms may have long periods of limited problems. When the restless legs syndrome and periodic limb movement disorder are the result of other conditions, such as anemia, usually there is no recurrence.

Diana, an eleven-year-old, was diagnosed with RLS and PLMD a year ago. Her parents were concerned about Diana, as her complaints were similar to those of her cousin and her grandfather, both of whom had been diagnosed with RLS. After testing, her doctor put her on an iron supplement. She also takes medication on some nights when her legs are really bothering her. It's made a major difference in how well she sleeps at night, and her grades in school have significantly improved. Her parents have even noticed smaller changes, such as being able to stay seated throughout dinner and no longer fidgeting when watching a movie.

15

Night Owls:
Delayed Sleep Phase Syndrome

Jonathon is in danger of flunking out of tenth grade because he has missed so many school days. In seventh and eighth grade he was enrolled in honors courses and doing well. However, in the past year Jonathon has been having more and more problems making it to school every day. In ninth grade, he was late most days, but this year, he can't seem to get to school at all. For the past month, he has basically given up going. The reason Jonathon has missed so much school is that he has problems falling asleep before 3:00 or 4:00 in the morning and then can't wake up in time for school. His parents desperately try to get him up, but instead he sleeps until noon. By that point, his parents have left for work and there is no way for Jonathon to get to school.

If you know an adolescent like Jonathon, you may have assumed that he was just being lazy or stubborn or is just a rebellious teenager. But in reality, Jonathan (and probably the teen you know) has a sleep disorder called *delayed sleep phase syndrome* (DSPS). Delayed sleep phase syndrome occurs when a person's internal sleep clock conflicts with the rest of his life's schedule needs. In this case, the clock is shifted (or "delayed") to a later bedtime, and wake time, than is compatible with normal activities such as getting up for school, going to work, and having a normal social life. So Jonathon is not being obstinate in refusing to get up for school in the morning; he literally can't. Delayed sleep phase syndrome is experienced by many teenagers and can have devastating effects, especially on school performance.

In delayed sleep phase syndrome, the sleep-wake cycle (internal clock) is generally delayed at least two hours later than what a normal bedtime would be (if there is such a thing in teenagers). For example, rather than falling asleep at 10:00 PM and waking at 7:00 AM, an adolescent with delayed sleep phase syndrome will not fall asleep until 2:00 AM and then has great difficulty waking up at 7:00 AM for school. If he is allowed to sleep until late in the morning, he will feel rested and can function well. Most children and adolescents with delayed sleep phase syndrome describe themselves as "night owls" and usually feel and function their best in the evening and nighttime hours. They usually get much less sleep on weekdays compared to weekends or holidays. Therefore, with DSPS it is the timing rather than the quality of sleep that is the problem.

As you can imagine, having delayed sleep phase syndrome, especially for children and adolescents who attend school, can cause significant problems, as they are unable to get up in time for school, often resulting in multiple school absences and tardiness.

DELAYED SLEEP PHASE SYNDROME

Delayed sleep phase syndrome is a significant and persistent shift in a child's or adolescent's internal clock that interferes with functioning, usually resulting in significant academic and behavior problems.

Adolescents with delayed sleep phase syndrome may complain of problems falling asleep or insomnia and have extreme difficulty waking up in the morning, even for things they really want to do (like hang out with friends). In order to cope, many adolescents with delayed sleep phase syndrome take long afternoon naps or catch up by sleeping longer on weekends and vacations. With delayed sleep phase syndrome, even highly motivated adolescents are unable to shift their sleep back to an earlier time without help.

Clues

A child or adolescent with delayed sleep phase syndrome often experiences the following symptoms:

- **A naturally late fall-asleep time.** The hallmark of DSPS is consistently not being able to fall asleep until very late, usually after midnight in adolescents, *even if the person really tries.*
- **Trouble falling asleep at a normal bedtime.** On nights that children or adolescents with delayed sleep phase syndrome try to go to sleep at a normal time, they are unable to do so. *However, if they were to go to bed at the time that they usually fall asleep, they have no problem.* Although, with effort, an adolescent with delayed sleep phase syndrome may temporarily fall asleep at an earlier time, there is a natural tendency to drift to a later bedtime.
- **Trouble getting up at a normal wake time.** As a result of falling asleep so late, many children and adolescents with delayed sleep phase syndrome are unable to wake up in the morning for school or other activities. This can result in many missed days or being late for school.
- **Complaints of insomnia.** When an adolescent with DSPS goes to bed early, he'll likely complain of insomnia, in that he can't fall asleep. It's like asking a well-rested adult to go to bed for the night at 6:00. You just can't do it. However, there will be no "insomnia" if bedtime occurs at the time your child usually falls asleep. This often occurs on weekends or school vacations.
- **No other sleep complaints.** Because the internal clock is simply shifted in children and adolescents with delayed sleep phase syndrome, once he is asleep your child will sleep well. In addition, on days he is able to sleep as long as he wishes, especially on weekends or holidays, he will not be sleepy during the day.
- **Daytime sleepiness.** Because of falling asleep so late and needing to get up early for school, your child may be very sleepy during the day. This may result in his taking a nap or falling asleep in school. He may also be moody and have problems paying attention.
- **Other daytime symptoms.** Some children and adolescents with delayed sleep phase syndrome experience problems with depression and other behavior problems as a result of the daytime sleepiness and the effects of missing school and social activities.

Other possible clues:

- **Bedtime resistance.** In younger children, bedtime resistance may occur. Children with an evening preference may have difficulty falling asleep at an age-appropriate bedtime, leading them to protest, make excuses, and outright refuse to go to bed.
- **Evening or night preference.** Given that most children and adolescents with DSPS are evening types, your child may feel and function at his best in the late afternoon, evening, or during the night. This may be the time that he does his best schoolwork or creative endeavors (such as art or writing).
- **Weekend oversleep.** To catch up from not getting enough sleep during the week, many adolescents will sleep until late morning or even early afternoon on the weekends. Your child may sleep for long hours, twelve hours or more, on weekends and vacations, especially during the first few days of the vacation.
- **Poor school performance.** Because adolescents with delayed sleep phase syndrome are often chronically sleep deprived, your child may perform poorly in school.
- **School tardiness and frequent absences.** Your child's sleep problem may lead to a downward spiral of missed school due to his being frequently late and absent, resulting in academic failure. Subsequently, he may begin to avoid going to school. In severe cases, a child or adolescent may give up going to school altogether.

How Common Is It?

Delayed sleep phase syndrome is experienced by about 5 to 10 percent of adolescents. Some younger children also have delayed sleep phase syndrome. It seems that boys are more likely to have delayed sleep phase syndrome than girls, but it is unclear why.

Causes

Delayed sleep phase syndrome usually develops during adolescence, but can start in childhood. Although the cause of delayed sleep phase syndrome is not completely known, it likely is an exaggerated reaction to the normal shift in sleep times that occurs during adolescence. After puberty, all adolescents have a shift in their internal clock of about two hours. In those with delayed sleep phase syndrome, the clock shifts even more. In addition, for children who already had a tendency to go to bed late, this normal two-hour shift will result in a significantly shifted internal clock. Thus, it is a shift of the brain's clock. Melatonin, which normally peaks at around 10:00 or 11:00 PM, will instead peak hours later. This major shift in the brain's clock often occurs at the same time that there is a change in your child's schedule, such as earlier start times in high school, which compounds the problem. Now, in addition to being unable to fall asleep until much later, your child also has to get up much earlier for school.

It's important to realize that this shift in sleep is not caused by deliberate behavior. Unfortunately, many adolescents with delayed sleep phase syndrome get labeled as noncompliant and truants. However, this disorder persists even when there are significant consequences, such as failing school or not being able to do things that the adolescent wants to do. Also, there is a high rate of relapse. Some evidence of a genetic link for this disorder has even appeared.

Making the Diagnosis

There is no definitive test for delayed sleep phase syndrome. The diagnosis is based on the description of the problem. Occasionally, an overnight sleep study (see page 187 for a description of this test) may be recommended to be sure that no other sleep disorder is present, such as obstructive sleep apnea (see chapter 13) or restless legs syndrome (see chapter 14).

Often an adolescent with DSPS has always been a lifelong "night owl." Ask your child questions about when he "feels best" during the day, such as what time he would prefer to go to bed, wake up in the morning, take a test, or play sports. Sample questions from a "morningness-eveningness" ("owl-lark") scale will help you determine if your child is prone to being an owl.

MORNINGNESS-EVENINGNESS SCALE

A few questions to determine if your child is more of a morning "lark" or an evening "owl."

1. If you were entirely free to plan your evening and had no commitments the next day, at what time would you choose to go to bed?
   - a.   8:00–9:00 PM
   - b.   9:00–10:15 PM
   - c.   10:15 PM–12:30 AM
   - d.   12:30–1:45 AM
   - e.   1:45–3:00 AM

2. For some reason you have gone to bed several hours later than normal, but there is no need to get up at a particular time the next morning. Which of the following is most likely to occur?
   - a.   Will wake up at the usual time and not fall asleep again
   - b.   Will wake up at the usual time and doze thereafter
   - c.   Will wake up at the usual time but will fall asleep again
   - d.   Will not wake up until later than usual

3. You have to take a two-hour test. If you were entirely free to choose, in which of the following periods would you prefer to take the test?
   - a.   8:00–10:00 AM
   - b.   11:00–1:30 PM
   - c.   3:00–5:00 PM
   - d.   7:00–9:00 PM

4. If you had no commitments the next day and were entirely free to plan your own day, what time would you get up?
   - a.   5:00–6:30 AM
   - b.   6:30–7:45 AM
   - c.   7:45–9:45 AM
   - d.   9:45–11:00 AM
   - e.   11:00 AM–12:00 PM

(Adapted from "A Self Assessment Questionnaire to Determine Morningness-Eveningness in Human Circadian Rhythms," by J.A. Horne and O. Ostberg, *International Journal of Chronobiology*, Vol. 4 (1976): 97–110.)

Keeping a daily sleep diary can be very helpful (see appendix A for a sample sleep diary). A sleep diary of a child with delayed sleep phase syndrome usually shows a late fall-asleep time that is usually about the same on most nights. Also, on weekends the child or adolescent typically goes to sleep even later and then sleeps in. The figure below shows a typical sleep diary of an adolescent with delayed sleep phase syndrome.

This chart shows what the overall pattern of sleep looks like for an adolescent with delayed sleep phase syndrome. S stands for sleep. The diary does not show exact times, just a basic pattern.

	2:00	3:00	4:00	5:00	6:00 ...	11:00	noon
Monday	S	S	S	S	S		
Tuesday	S	S	S	S	S		
Wednesday	S	S	S	S	S		
Thursday	S	S	S	S	S		
Friday		S	S	S	S	S	S
Saturday		S	S	S	S	S	S
Sunday	S	S	S	S	S		
Monday	S	S	S	S	S		

What Else Could It Be?

There are other factors that can cause your child to have problems falling asleep at night, not fall asleep until late at night, have problems waking up in the morning, and/or be sleepy during the day.

- **Insomnia.** Problems falling asleep at night may be the result of insomnia (see chapter 11). One clear differentiation between DSPS and insomnia is that children and adolescents with delayed sleep phase syndrome have little or no problem falling asleep if they go to bed at the time they normally fall asleep. Children and adolescents with insomnia, however, have problems falling asleep no matter what time they go to bed. They also do not have a consistent time that they almost always fall asleep.

- **Restless legs syndrome.** Restless legs syndrome often leads to a child or adolescent taking a long time to fall asleep at night. In addition, a child will have uncomfortable feelings in her legs. See chapter 14 for a complete description of restless legs syndrome.

- **Bad sleep habits.** Poor sleep habits, including keeping an erratic sleep schedule and using caffeine or other substances, may result in complaints of difficulty falling asleep. Some adolescents with DSPS also develop sleep habits that are ultimately counterproductive (such as lying in bed awake for long periods) in an attempt to fix their sleep problem. However, adolescents with delayed sleep phase syndrome still have trouble falling asleep early, even after establishing an appropriate sleep schedule and developing good sleep habits.

- **Being a night owl.** Although a preference for evening hours ("night owl") puts a child at risk for developing delayed sleep phase syndrome, it is not the same. "Eveningness" does not have the same intractable quality and persistence, and does not result in major school and behavior problems.

- **Lifestyle issues.** Staying up late at night to watch television, instant message, or talk on the phone with friends often leads to later bedtime times and thus a more difficult time getting up in the morning for school. Get rid of the television, unplug the computer, and turn off the phone. That should solve the problem.

- **School avoidance or school refusal.** Some children and adolescents with a delayed sleep phase actually have problems with school avoidance or school refusal. These children, who are usually depressed or anxious to begin with or may have social or learning problems, often start out by missing a week or two of school as a result of an illness, travel, or for family reasons. They then have a hard time catching up on schoolwork and may avoid returning to school. In many cases, the stated reason for not attending school is a physical one (headaches, abdominal pain, chronic fatigue), and sometimes it is a sleep problem. These kids fall asleep late and refuse to get up or can't wake up in the morning on school days (often in spite of drastic measures by parents, such as pouring cold water on them or literally dragging them out of bed). On weekends and holidays (non–school days), however, they often get up without a problem. The longer they go without attending school, the more difficult it is to break the cycle, and, in severe cases, adolescents may end up dropping out of school altogether.

The major difference between DSPS and a sleep problem associated with school avoidance is that kids with DSPS want to get better and will try anything to improve their sleep, while the school-avoidant child or teenager will do everything to sabotage getting better (sometimes without realizing it), because she *really doesn't want to go back to school.* The key is to recognize the "psychosomatic" (meaning a combination of physical and psychological issues) nature of the problem and to get counseling for these kids, because treating the sleep problem alone will not address the real issues.

- **Psychiatric problems.** Teens with depression, bipolar disorder, or an anxiety disorder can also have problems falling asleep at night and getting up in the morning. Your doctor or school psychologist can help determine whether your child is having any of these problems.
- **Substance use.** Given the high prevalence of drug and alcohol use by teenagers, it is important to determine whether your adolescent is taking part. If your he is having problems with alcohol or drug use, he won't have a consistent sleep schedule as is seen with delayed sleep phase syndrome.

Sleep Solutions

Delayed sleep phase syndrome is a difficult disorder to treat and requires significant effort on the part of both you and your child. Thus, for treatment to be successful, your child has to be very motivated. The goal of treatment is to retrain the internal clock to follow a more regular schedule. Making the initial shift in the sleep-wake cycle is easy; however, keeping it there is much harder. Treatment involves changes in sleep habits and a shift in the brain's clock. Sometimes medication and/or bright light therapy are helpful.

- **Have good sleep habits.** Good sleep habits are especially important for children and adolescents with delayed sleep phase syndrome. These habits should include a regular sleep schedule of going to bed and waking up at the same time every day; avoidance of caffeine, smoking, and other drugs; a bedroom environment that is cool, quiet, and comfortable; a bedtime routine that is calm and sleep-inducing; and avoidance of all stimulating activities before bed, such as computer games and television. (See chapter 6 for more information on good sleep practices for your child.)
- **Beat the clock.** Treatment for delayed sleep phase syndrome involves systematically shifting the internal clock. There are two ways to go about it, either advancing or delaying bedtime on successive nights.

  - **Phase advancement.** Phase advancement involves moving the bedtime earlier by fifteen minutes on each successive night. If your adolescent usually falls asleep at 12:30, then bedtime is set for 12:15 for one or two nights, 12:00 for one or two nights, and so on. If your adolescent also sleeps in every morning, shift his wake time using the exact same schedule.

SAMPLE PHASE ADVANCEMENT SCHEDULE

	Bedtime	Wake
Before	1:30 AM	10:00 AM
Treatment night 1	1:15	9:45
Treatment night 2	1:00	9:30
Treatment night 3	12:45	9:15
Treatment night 4	12:30	9:00
Treatment night 5	12:15	8:45
Treatment night 14	10:30 PM	6:30 AM

- **Phase delay (chronotherapy).** Phase delay should be chosen if your adolescent's naturally occurring bedtime is three or more hours later than desired. For this scenario, bedtime is delayed by two to three hours on each successive night. For example, if your adolescent usually falls asleep at 2:00 AM, delay bedtime until 4:00 AM on night one, 6:00 AM on night two, and so on until the desired bedtime is reached (for example, 10:30 PM). Given that it is much easier for the body to adjust to a later bedtime than an earlier one, it is often recommended to delay bedtime rather than try to advance it. Adolescents are often compliant during the first phase of this treatment because of the perception that they are being allowed to stay up later each day. If possible, this method should be timed to coincide with a school vacation to avoid missing school during the time your child will be scheduled to sleep during the day.

SAMPLE PHASE DELAY SCHEDULE		
	Bedtime	Wake time
Before	4:30 AM	12:30 PM
Treatment night 1	7:30	3:30
Treatment night 2	10:30	6:30
Treatment night 3	1:30	9:30
Treatment night 4	4:30	12:30
Treatment night 5	7:30	3:30
Treatment night 6	10:30	6:30
Treatment night 14	10:30 PM	6:30 AM

- **Stick with it.** Once the desired bedtime is reached, your child must stick with it on a nightly basis. Even one late night of studying or socializing can return the internal clock to being delayed. Thus, all it takes to undo all achievements is one weekend or vacation in which old habits are resumed. Once the new schedule is firmly entrenched, in a month or two, an occasional late night is permitted, but your child should not be allowed to sleep more than one or two hours later than his usual weekday wake time.

- **Light up the morning.** Have your teenager eat breakfast in a sunny place in the house, open all the shades in the morning, and don't let him wear sunglasses when he is heading off to school. Exposure to bright light in the morning will help reset his body's internal clock to an earlier time. Bright light therapy can also be helpful. It involves exposure to bright light in the morning for approximately twenty to thirty minutes. A special light box can be purchased for this purpose. Talk with your doctor or a sleep specialist about how to get one of these light boxes and how best to use it.

- **Stay in the dark.** By the same token, adolescents with DSPS should avoid bright light at night so their melatonin is able to turn on at bedtime.

MOTIVATION IS KEY TO SUCCESSFUL TREATMENT

An adolescent needs to be highly motivated to be successful in realigning his sleep schedule and maintaining the change. A well-developed plan is essential. Working out a contract and having everyone agree to the changes that need to be made is crucial.

- **Talk with the school.** Because children and teenagers with DSPS may have been labeled as lazy or truant, it is very important to help school officials understand that your child has a real, physical sleep problem that needs to be treated (your may want to enlist your doctor's help in explaining this). And since the treatment sometimes involves temporarily missing school while the sleep cycle is being adjusted, it's critical to have the school's support. That is not to say the school should not hold you or your child accountable for seeking treatment or give permission for him to be late every day. A compromise that balances your child's sleep needs and school responsibilities should be worked out. In addition, because many of these kids have fallen behind in their schoolwork, a detailed plan should be developed so that he can catch up within a reasonable period of time. This can help lessen a child's anxiety about returning to school and decrease the chances that he will develop school avoidance.

- **Encourage responsibility.** Often long-standing battles exist between children with DSPS and their parents over going to bed and getting up in the morning. Try to diminish the fighting by having your child take responsibility for his sleep schedule. Another issue that can sometimes compromise treatment success is the social aspect of DSPS. Your child may need help in coming up with an explanation to his classmates about why she has missed so much school ("saving face"). Other kids may think she has been getting away with something by coming in late so often, and your child may need some guidance from you about how to handle the situation and take charge.

16

"I'm So Sleepy": Narcolepsy

Christopher is sixteen years old and has frequently fallen asleep in school during the past year. Last week, though, he fell asleep while driving, which scared both him and his parents. Although Christopher gets plenty of sleep at night, he just can't seem to stay awake during the day.

Narcolepsy is a chronic sleep disorder that involves an uncontrollable and overwhelming feeling of sleepiness. Although narcolepsy affects mostly adults, symptoms can first appear in adolescence and even during childhood. Unfortunately, most children and adolescents who have signs of narcolepsy are misdiagnosed or never get evaluated at all. Therefore, they miss out on the opportunity to start appropriate treatment. Although narcolepsy is a relatively rare condition, its impact on a child or adolescent's life can be dramatic.

The daytime sleepiness that is typically seen in narcolepsy is not just dozing off on long car rides or nodding off in class once in a while. People with narcolepsy usually fall asleep frequently throughout the day, generally for short periods of ten to twenty minutes. The urge to fall sleep is also extremely powerful—so much so that it is often described as "irresistible"—even when the person fights to stay awake. These daytime sleep episodes are also called *sleep attacks,* suggesting just how swift and stealthy they can be. And, most importantly, this profound sleepiness occurs *despite getting a good night's sleep the night before.*

NARCOLEPSY

Narcolepsy is a relatively rare chronic neurological disorder and causes significant problems during the day. The hallmark of narcolepsy is excessive daytime sleepiness. Other symptoms include cataplexy, hypnagogic hallucinations, and sleep paralysis.

Clues

The symptoms of narcolepsy can appear all at once or, more commonly, they can develop slowly over many years. The four most common symptoms are *excessive daytime sleepiness, cataplexy, sleep paralysis,* and *hypnagogic hallucinations* (that's a mouthful!). Although these symptoms may sound rather bizarre and seem to have little in common, they are all related in some way to the underlying sleep-wake abnormalities that occur in narcolepsy. Basically, people with narcolepsy suddenly exhibit certain features of sleep (particularly REM or "dream" sleep) while they are otherwise wide-awake. For example, a prominent feature of REM sleep is a loss of normal body muscle tone and movement (this basically prevents us from acting out our dreams). Cataplexy and sleep paralysis involve a similar loss of muscle tone, but this time it occurs while the person is awake. Hypnagogic hallucinations are really dream fragments that show up or "intrude" as the person is falling asleep (rather than waiting politely for REM sleep to occur).

- **Excessive daytime sleepiness.** For most children and adolescents with narcolepsy, daytime sleepiness is the first symptom to appear, and for many it remains the only symptom for years. Children and adolescents with narcolepsy often feel easily tired or tired all the time. They tend to fall asleep not only at times when many other people feel sleepy (such as while watching a movie or during a dull lecture), but also when most people would be wide-awake (such as in the middle of a conversation or at the dinner table). People with narcolepsy may also fall asleep at unusual times (even while standing up!) or under dangerous circumstances (driving a car). Most narcoleptics describe these naps as "refreshing," which means that they seem to relieve the feelings of sleepiness, at least temporarily. *Microsleeps,* which are extremely brief (several seconds) sleep periods, may also occur. A child with narcolepsy is usually unaware of these microsleeps, and parents and teachers may interpret such periods as daydreaming or just not paying attention.

- **Cataplexy.** Cataplexy is a sudden, brief loss of muscle tone that is triggered by a strong emotion, especially laughter. It can also happen after feeling angry, sad, or surprised. Symptoms of cataplexy can range from a brief feeling of weakness in the knees or a drooping of the head to a complete collapse on the floor. During these episodes, your child will be completely conscious and will remember the event. These episodes can last from seconds to minutes and may occur from several times a day to just a few times per year. Cataplexy is rarely the first symptom of narcolepsy, but often develops within the first year of the daytime sleepiness (although sometimes not until twenty years later!). About 60 percent of children and adolescents with narcolepsy experience cataplexy.
- **Hypnagogic hallucinations.** These are incredibly vivid, dreamlike experiences that occur when your child is falling asleep or just waking up in the morning. These images are often scary, such as of strange animals or prowlers, and are particularly frightening because a child is awake but has no control over them. They are difficult to distinguish from reality. Hypnagogic hallucinations are reported by 50 to 70 percent of adults with narcolepsy. It's important to realize that children and adolescents who don't have narcolepsy may also occasionally experience hypnagogic hallucinations, especially when they are sleep deprived.
- **Sleep paralysis.** Sleep paralysis is a feeling of being paralyzed or unable to move for a few minutes either when falling asleep or just after waking up. Sleep paralysis may occur at the same time as hypnagogic hallucinations. Imagine thinking you see a strange creature in the corner of the room as you are lying in bed, and yet you can't move a muscle to cry out or run away. This should give you some sense of how frightening these experiences can be. Luckily, touching someone when he has sleep paralysis usually makes it

end. Sleep paralysis occurs in 40 to 65 percent of narcoleptics and, as with hypnagogic hallucinations, also is occasionally experienced by children and adolescents who don't have narcolepsy.

COMMON SYMPTOMS OF NARCOLEPSY

- Excessive daytime sleepiness (falling asleep in school or at inappropriate times)
- Short refreshing naps
- Sleep disruption
- Hypnagogic hallucinations
- Sleep paralysis
- Automatic behaviors
- Inattention, poor concentration, distractibility
- Academic problems
- Social problems

Other possible symptoms of narcolepsy include:

- **Automatic behavior.** Automatic behavior is the performance of familiar, routine, or boring tasks without being aware of doing them or remembering them later on (being on "auto-pilot"). This is also the result of sleep sneaking into the middle of wakefulness. Sometimes a child may fall asleep in the middle of an activity and continue with the activity but not recall having done so when he wakes up. An example of automatic behavior is writing a page of nonsense in the middle of doing homework.
- **Poor sleep.** Although you would expect that a child with narcolepsy would sleep soundly at night, sleep is often disrupted. Your child may wake up during the night, making the daytime sleepiness even worse.
- **Vivid dreams.** Your child may have very vivid dreams. Furthermore, because people with narcolepsy, unlike the rest of us, go immediately into dream or REM sleep as soon as they fall asleep,

lots of dreaming may occur at the beginning of the night. For the same reason, your child may dream even during short daytime naps.

- **Poor academic performance.** Given the likelihood of falling asleep in school, many children with narcolepsy begin to do poorly in school. In addition, children and adolescents with narcolepsy may be labeled as lazy, inattentive, and be viewed as behavior problems.
- **Daytime problems.** Some children and adolescents with narcolepsy have problems paying attention and difficulty concentrating. They may be easily distracted. This is related to being sleepy. There may also be concerns about their behavior, such as hyperactivity. Some children even have significant social problems and trouble keeping up with friends.

THE GREAT MASQUERADER

The symptoms of narcolepsy are frequently misdiagnosed as psychiatric or behavioral disorders, including ADHD, depression, and even psychosis.

How Common Is It?

Narcolepsy is quite rare. In the United States approximately three to sixteen per ten thousand people have narcolepsy (compare that to about three thousand per ten thousand children who resist going to bed or wake up at night). In addition, most people with narcolepsy do not get diagnosed for many years after they first develop symptoms, and some are never diagnosed. It is estimated that as many as two hundred thousand Americans have narcolepsy, but that less than one-quarter of them have been diagnosed with the disorder.

- **Gender.** Narcolepsy affects boys and girls equally.
- **Ethnicity:** Narcolepsy is more common in certain ethnic groups, with the disorder found in one out of six hundred people in Japan, compared to one in four thousand in North America and Europe. Interestingly, only one in five hundred thousand people in Israel have narcolepsy.
- **Age of onset:** Most people with narcolepsy develop symptoms after

puberty, starting sometime between the ages of fifteen and thirty, but symptoms can develop in younger children as well. One study found that 16 percent of adults with narcolepsy described having symptoms before the age of ten; however only about 4 percent of narcoleptics are diagnosed before the age of fifteen. The average time between onset of symptoms and diagnosis is ten to fifteen years.

- **Family history:** A family history of narcolepsy or excessive daytime sleepiness is more commonly found in children with narcolepsy symptoms than in the general population.

Causes

In the last several years, there have been a number of exciting breakthroughs in our understanding of what causes narcolepsy. Narcolepsy appears to involve a problem with the part of the central nervous system that controls sleep and wakefulness. Recent discoveries suggest that a neurotransmitter (brain chemical) called *orexin/hypocretin* is likely to be involved. Orexin/hypocretin is reduced or absent in many, but not all, people with narcolepsy. An autoimmune problem, possibly triggered by a virus, may also play a role in causing narcolepsy.

Narcolepsy also often runs in families, but many people with narcolepsy do not have relatives who are affected. Children of narcoleptics have an increased risk for developing narcolepsy. Their risk is 1 percent, which is forty times that of the general population. In addition, it is estimated that 8 to 12 percent of people diagnosed with narcolepsy have a close family relative, such as a parent or a sibling, with the disorder. Furthermore, up to 40 percent of people have a family member with a history of excessive daytime sleepiness.

Gregory is seventeen years old and was recently diagnosed with narcolepsy. It had always been a known fact that his grandfather was very sleepy. He was notorious for falling asleep at family gatherings, even at his own daughter's wedding. Gregory's cousin also had a problem with falling asleep all the time and didn't join the military because he was worried that he would get in trouble for falling asleep on duty.

Genetics, however, does not account for all cases of narcolepsy. For example, there have been cases where one twin of a set of identical twins had narcolepsy and the other did not. If narcolepsy were purely genetic, both identical twins would have it. Thus, there are clearly other factors (environment, infections) that may be involved. For example, one study of over eight hundred people with narcolepsy from the United States, Canada, and France found that those born in March were more likely to develop narcolepsy, while those born in September had the lowest risk!

In general, though, most cases of narcolepsy are considered "idiopathic," meaning that there is no known reason for why it developed.

Making the Diagnosis

The diagnosis of narcolepsy requires an overnight sleep study, followed the next day by a special type of sleep study called a *multiple sleep latency test* (MSLT). The purpose of the overnight sleep study is to evaluate whether other sleep problems might be present that could possibly explain the symptoms and be making your child sleepy, such as obstructive sleep apnea (see chapter 13) or periodic limb movements (see chapter 14). The MSLT is the best test available for documenting the extent of daytime sleepiness that a person has. The day after the overnight sleep study, the patient is given a set number (four or five) of opportunities to try to fall asleep. These nap opportunities are twenty minutes long and are spaced out at intervals of every two hours. Whether or not your child falls asleep during each nap opportunity and, if so, how long it takes him to fall asleep are recorded. In addition, the presence of REM sleep during any of the naps is also noted, as this is a marker for narcolepsy. However, especially in children and adolescents, the initial studies are often inconclusive, and several overnight sleep studies over a period of several months or several years might be required in order to make a definitive diagnosis.

What Else Could It Be?

There are many other causes of daytime sleepiness. You should always consider the following list of possibilities, especially given how rare narcolepsy is in the population.

- **Chronic sleep deprivation and erratic sleep-wake schedules.** Not getting enough sleep is the number one reason that a child or adolescent is very sleepy during the day. Be sure to check chapter 3 to see how much sleep your child should be getting. If he is not getting enough sleep, move bedtime earlier and work out schedules so that he can get the sleep that he needs. Also, going to bed and waking up at different times every day (classic of college students) can lead to significant daytime sleepiness. So make sure your child keeps a regular schedule and gets enough sleep at night.
- **Sleep need.** There are some children and adolescents who simply need more sleep than others. Surprisingly to many, people with narcolepsy typically do not sleep more hours than average at night. It's not that they literally need more sleep than others; it's just that they get very sleepy at many times throughout the day.
- **Other sleep disorders.** Anything that disrupts your child's sleep during the night will make her feel sleepy the next day. These sleep disorders may include obstructive sleep apnea (see chapter 13), restless legs syndrome (see chapter 14), and periodic limb movement disorder (see chapter 14). Be sure to consider any of these more common sleep disorders that also lead to daytime sleepiness.
- **Idiopathic hypersomnia.** There's that word again, "idiopathic," that basically means we haven't yet figured out what causes the problem. People with idiopathic hypersomnia look very much like people with narcolepsy in terms of daytime sleepiness, but they do not have the other symptoms (such as cataplexy). This is also a lifelong disorder, and, although rare, can have a very significant effect on daytime functioning and may be quite difficult to treat.
- **Kleine-Levin syndrome.** Another rare disorder is Kleine-Levin syndrome, which occurs almost exclusively in adolescent boys and is believed to be related to a dysfunction in an area of the brain called the hypothalamus. Kleine-Levin syndrome involves excessive sleepiness that occurs in periods of several days to weeks, rather than on a daily basis as it does in narcolepsy. People who experience this syndrome are basically normal in between the sleepy periods. Children or adolescents with Kleine-Levin usually

have other symptoms of hypothalamus dysfunction during these periods, including overeating and inappropriate sexual behavior.

- **Menstrual cycle–related sleepiness.** This rare cause of episodic (occurring at regular intervals) sleepiness in adolescent girls and young women seems to be related to changes in hormone levels during the menstrual cycle. The most severe sleepiness seems to occur just before the start of the menstrual period and is sometimes treated with birth control pills.
- **Psychiatric disorders/depression.** Psychiatric disorders, especially depression, should be considered if your child or adolescent is significantly sleepy during the day and also has other symptoms of depression, such as lack of appetite and lack of interest in activities he used to enjoy (such as playing with friends or going to the movies). Your doctor should be able to help evaluate for any of these types of problems.
- **Other causes.** There are many other causes for being sleepy during the day, such as a side effect of a medication (see chapter 19) or a previous illness, such as mononucleosis. Sleepiness can also occur following an accident, such as a head injury or a concussion. It can also be related to alcohol or drug use in an adolescent.

Sleep Solutions

Narcolepsy cannot be cured, but its symptoms can usually be controlled so that a child or adolescent with narcolepsy can lead a normal life. Treatment usually includes the following:

- **Medications.** Medications are often prescribed for narcolepsy. Usually a medication is recommended to help combat the daytime sleepiness, such as a stimulant, including Ritalin, Dexadrine, Concerta, or Adderall. There is also a newer medication, Provigil, which is prescribed specifically for the treatment of daytime sleepiness in narcolepsy. People with cataplexy require a different type of medication, usually a drug that decreases or suppresses REM sleep. These medications include several different types of antidepressants.

- **Skip the Starbucks.** Caffeine should be avoided, especially in the late afternoon and evening, so that your child's nighttime sleep is not disturbed. It is better to have your child take a medication, rather than use caffeine, to stay awake during the day.
- **Develop good sleep habits.** Excellent sleep habits are essential for children and adolescents with narcolepsy (see chapter 6). Have your child keep a strict sleep schedule. Your child should go to bed and get up at the same time every day. Also, it's crucial that your child gets adequate sleep every night.
- **Take a nap.** Have your child take a short nap once or twice a day. These naps can help control the daytime sleepiness, along with a medication. Speak to your child's teacher or school nurse about ways to incorporate a fifteen- to thirty-minute nap into your child's school day.
- **Change your child's lifestyle.** Your child will also be greatly helped by changes in his lifestyle.
  - Increase physical activity; avoid boring or repetitive tasks.
  - Avoid activities that can be dangerous, such as driving, swimming, or cooking, except during times when you know your child will be alert. All adolescents with narcolepsy must be well treated prior to allowing them to drive.
- **Don't keep it a secret.** Tell others about your child's sleep problem. Be sure to let others know that your child has narcolepsy, especially teachers. It's common for the sleepiness to be mistaken for laziness, boredom, or lack of ability, especially if she is falling asleep in school. Small adjustments in the classroom, such as being seated in the front of the class and being chosen to run classroom errands, can make a tremendous difference in your child's school performance. Encourage your child to tell her friends, and share the information with the parents of your child's friends. Again, you don't want your child to be misunderstood when she falls asleep at unusual times. And, of course, let relatives such as grandparents, aunts and uncles, and cousins, and especially brothers and sisters know about the narcolepsy and help them to understand the condition.

PART FOUR: SLEEP ISSUES

17

Why Johnny Can't Pay Attention . . . or Sleep!: Sleep and ADHD

Blake is seven years old and is repeating first grade. He can't sit still and has problems paying attention. His parents say he has been like this for as long as they can remember. He was recently diagnosed with ADHD, and his parents and teachers have seen some positive changes since they started treatment. However, his parents are still having major problems at night. Blake often refuses to get into bed, and even after they turn out the lights, it can be hours before he is finally asleep. Both of his parents are exhausted and dread what they call the "beastly hours" of the day.

Attention-deficit/hyperactivity disorder (ADHD) is the most commonly diagnosed psychiatric disorder in children, affecting about 5–10 percent of children in the United States. Symptoms of ADHD usually develop before age seven and include difficulty paying attention and distractibility, problems staying on task, and difficulty completing schoolwork. Children with ADHD can pay attention to some tasks, but usually not unless they are very motivated or interested in something, such as television or video games. In addition, they often have difficulty shifting their attention from one activity to another and concentrating when there are distractions. They may also have problems focusing on what is most important (seeing the "forest" instead of the "trees"). Many children with ADHD are also hyperactive and have impulsive behaviors, such as talking out of turn and interrupting. They may not be able to stay seated and may fidget all the time. Older children and adolescents often develop more subtle impairments in what is called *executive functioning,* such as having problems with being organized and complex thinking skills. For the majority of children who are diagnosed with ADHD, the condition is lifelong.

That is what ADHD is. This is what ADHD is not. It is not a just a catchall phrase for any kid who misbehaves a little in the classroom or acts up for grandma. It is not merely a label used by a society that expects perfection in all its members, including its youngest. It is not a disease dreamed up by the medical community and the pharmaceutical industry in order to "drug our kids." And it is not the result of bad (permissive) parenting, too much TV, too much sugar, too little sugar, allergies, or artificial anything. In reality, ADHD is a complex disorder that results from "miswiring" of a number of important brain centers that control attention, activity, and behavior. It does involve changes in the normal levels of brain chemicals (neurotransmitters) in these specific areas of the central nervous system. And these differences in the ADHD brain are most likely programmed into our genetic makeup from day one.

Diagnosis. There is considerable controversy these days, as the previous discussion suggests, about the over-diagnosis of ADHD. In all likelihood, ADHD is probably *under-diagnosed* (particularly in girls) as often as it is incorrectly identified. So how do you as a parent protect your fidgety or inattentive child from being mislabeled as having ADHD (or, alternatively, not having ADHD)? First, the diagnosis of ADHD should be made by a doctor or mental health provider following a *comprehensive evaluation.* This evaluation should include a review of ADHD symptoms across time and across different settings, including at school, at home, and in social situations. It is also important to rule out or eliminate other possible causes for the ADHD symptoms, such as medical or other psychiatric problems. As much as we wish there were one simple test for ADHD, there is not, but psychological and educational testing may be helpful in supporting the diagnosis and evaluating for possible learning disabilities. The key here is to have your child evaluated by a professional who is experienced, comes well-recommended, and *is someone you trust to help you make decisions that are in the best interest of your child and your family.*

Treatment. The most common treatments for ADHD include the following:

- **Behavioral management.** Behavioral strategies are the foundation for managing not only the ADHD symptoms but also any related problem behaviors, such as aggression or defiance, both at home and at school. There are many excellent parenting books available on this topic. You may also want to consider behavioral management counseling, which can be extremely helpful in problem-solving and in developing an individualized approach.

- **Classroom accommodations.** Examples of classroom modifications and school-based accommodations that can benefit children with ADHD include being seated in the front of the classroom near the teacher, modified homework assignments, and allowing a child to use a computer to complete written assignments. The most important thing you can do is to be an advocate for your child within the school system. Although occasionally this requires an in-your-face approach, most of the time schools will work with you if you stay involved and work together as a team.

- **Individual and family counseling.** Many children with ADHD benefit from counseling to address family issues, improve social skills, and boost self-esteem.

- **Medication.** Although in some circles the use of medication for children with ADHD has gotten a bad rap (e.g., www.ritalinkills.com), it can be a miracle worker for many kids. The right medication can be extremely helpful in reducing hyperactive behavior and improving impulse control and attention. Studies have shown that use of ADHD medications results in long-term gains in social skills and improvements in self-esteem. And contrary to what you might have heard, children with ADHD who are successfully treated with medication are less likely to become drug and alcohol users as young adults. Of course, finding the right medication for your child, one that provides good control of ADHD symptoms without problematic side effects, frequently involves some degree of trial and error. This process can be understandably frustrating for parents and children, but it is necessary in order to provide the most effective and safest treatment.

Other issues. It is also important to note that the majority of children with ADHD have other emotional, behavioral, and learning problems in addition to the ADHD. These may include depression, anxiety, and oppositional defiant behaviors. It's important to recognize these other kinds of problems, because standard ADHD treatments may not work as well or may not address all of the symptoms.

ADHD and Sleep

There are several very important ways in which ADHD and sleep (and sleepiness) appear to be related. First, there is a great deal of overlap between the symptoms of ADHD, such as difficulty concentrating and hyperactivity, and behaviors associated with not getting enough sleep. In other words, sleepiness resulting from sleep problems in children may be impossible to distinguish from symptoms of ADHD. This means that some children with a sleep disorder may be incorrectly diagnosed as having ADHD.

Second, many children and adolescents with ADHD complain of chronic difficulties with disturbed sleep. They often have problems falling asleep, staying asleep, and restless sleep. These sleep issues often start in early childhood. In fact, 25 to 50 percent of children and adolescents with ADHD report sleep problems. Not only are sleep problems common in ADHD, but they can also exacerbate the ADHD symptoms.

Finally, some intriguing research findings suggest there is a relationship between brain centers that control attention and behavior and those that regulate sleep and wakefulness. This indicates that these two processes may be linked.

Sleepy, Dopey, and Grumpy

Every parent knows what an overtired child is like—cranky, fussy, whiny, short-tempered, difficult to manage, and generally unpleasant to be around. In addition, somewhat paradoxically, parents frequently describe sleepy children as "hyper," "wound-up," and "out of control."

Children who have not gotten enough sleep or are overtired show a range of behaviors. As with adult cases, some of these behaviors are typically associated with being sleepy, such as yawning, rubbing their eyes, nodding, or resting their head on a desk (less common in children). Children, however, may also act out when they are tired, becoming more impulsive, hyperactive, and aggressive (more common, especially in younger children). Sleepiness can also result in learning and attention problems that may be seen by both parents and teachers. These behaviors include problems with processing information, difficulty focusing and maintaining attention, slower response time, less flexible and creative thinking, poor reasoning and judgment, and memory problems. As you can see, these mood, behavioral, and cognitive problems that are a result of sleepiness are practically a carbon copy of those associated with ADHD. Thus, the challenge is trying to determine what parts of your child's problems are due to ADHD and what parts may be due to not getting enough sleep or getting a poor night's sleep.

The Great Pretenders: Sleep Disorders That Masquerade as ADHD

Some children with ADHD may actually have a sleep disorder that causes at least some of their behavior and attention problems. The most common sleep disorders that may "cause" ADHD symptoms are obstructive sleep apnea (see chapter 13), restless legs syndrome, and periodic limb movement disorder (see chapter 14).

A SLEEP PROBLEM . . . NOT ADHD

Basically, if your child has any of the following symptoms, you should get him checked for a sleep problem:
- Loud snoring
- Gasping
- Breathing pauses
- Restless sleep
- Kicking movements
- Major difficulties falling asleep and/or staying asleep

- **Obstructive sleep apnea.** Children with obstructive sleep apnea often have problems with attention, memory, and higher-level executive functions. They may also have problems with impulsivity, hyperactivity, aggression, and conduct problems. Sound familiar? It should; these symptoms are practically identical to those seen in a child with ADHD. Symptoms of anxiety, depression, and poor school performance are also more common in children with sleep apnea.

Studies have suggested that as many as 25 percent of children diagnosed with ADHD may have symptoms of sleep apnea. In addition, snoring is three times more common in children with ADHD. Finally, and perhaps most telling, a number of studies have looked at behavior and cognitive functioning in children following treatment for sleep apnea (this usually involves removing the tonsils and adenoids). In these children, significant improvements were seen in daytime sleepiness, behavior, attention, learning, and school performance after treatment. Therefore, every child who is being evaluated for ADHD should be screened (and treated, if necessary) for symptoms of sleep apnea. (See chapter 13 for a list of symptoms of sleep apnea and what to look for in your child).

- **Restless legs syndrome (RLS) and periodic limb movement disorder (PLMD).** Although less common in children, these two disorders may also be associated with behavior and attention problems. In one study, for example, almost two-thirds of children evaluated for ADHD had RLS/PLMD. Another study of children with ADHD seen in a pediatric sleep clinic found PLMD in more than a third of the children. Treatment of these sleep problems not only improved sleep, but it also improved the ADHD-like behaviors. Chapter 14 provides complete information on these two sleep disorders.

So what should you do with all this information? Well, first, because doctors aren't always good about asking parents the right questions about sleep, it's important for you to recognize the possible relationship between sleep problems and ADHD. Second, talk with your child's doctor about any possible symptoms of sleep disorders, such as snoring or very restless sleep.

Belinda was concerned about her daughter Tiffany. Tiffany had been diagnosed with ADHD two years ago when she was seven. She was doing better, but her mother noticed that she didn't seem to sleep well and was always tired the next day. Belinda asked her doctor to have Tiffany checked out for a sleep problem. Tiffany ended up having sleep apnea, and the doctors removed her tonsils and adenoids. After the surgery, Tiffany's behavior was dramatically improved, although not perfect.

Even if the sleep problem is not the only cause of your child's ADHD symptoms, treatment of the problem will help. So don't be afraid to ask questions and volunteer information; it may avoid unnecessary or inappropriate treatment!

Causes of Sleep Problems in Children with ADHD

There are many possible causes of sleep problems in children with ADHD. For example, one of the common side effects of ADHD medications—particularly stimulant medications such as Ritalin, Concerta, Dexedrine, and Adderall—is sleep problems, especially problems with falling asleep. As many parents of children with ADHD are well aware, stimulant medications may have a rebound effect when they wear off at the end of the day, resulting in an increase in ADHD (hyperactivity, impulsivity) symptoms. These, in turn, may lead to difficulty in settling and falling asleep at bedtime. In some cases, a late-day dose of stimulant medication to avoid this rebound can solve the problem.

In addition to medication effects, other emotional and behavioral conditions that frequently accompany ADHD, such as oppositional defiant disorder, depression, and anxiety, can affect sleep. For example, children who are oppositional may resist and struggle at bedtime. Children with anxiety disorders may have difficulty falling asleep at bedtime or falling back to sleep during the night as a result of multiple fears and worries that surface during the night. Sleep problems are also common in other childhood anxiety disorders, such as obsessive-compulsive disorder and in children and adolescents with depression. Three-quarters of adolescents with major depression report some degree of insomnia, and almost a third of them describe severe sleep difficulties. Settling down at bedtime and night wakings may also be related to other conditions that frequently coexist with ADHD, such as sensory integration disorder. And children with Tourette's syndrome may have sleep difficulties related to tics occurring during sleep.

Is Sleep in Children with ADHD Different?

There is little question that parents frequently report sleep complaints in their children with ADHD. In fact, restless and disturbed sleep was once considered to be one of the criteria used for making the diagnosis of ADHD (although this is no longer the case). However, much of the research on whether some or all children with ADHD sleep differently (or less well, or not as much) compared to other children has resulted in contradictory findings.

Studies of children with ADHD that have used questionnaires have almost universally reported a higher prevalence of sleep problems, including difficulty falling asleep, night wakings, and restless sleep. On the other hand, most of the studies that have used more objective measures, such as overnight sleep studies or *actigraphy* (which uses a wristwatch-like device to measure and store data about movement), have largely failed to find differences between children with and without ADHD. In particular, there is no scientific evidence that children with ADHD need less sleep than other children do.

There are several notable exceptions to this general lack of differences between the sleep of children with and without ADHD. For one, activity or restlessness in the sleep of children with ADHD seems to be greater compared to other children. In addition, there appears to be more variability in sleep patterns from one night to the next in children with ADHD. What these differences actually mean is not yet clear, but they do raise further questions about whether there are distinct features of sleep in children with ADHD.

So why is there such inconsistency between what parents report about the sleep of their children with ADHD and research findings? There are a number of possible explanations. One possibility is that one night's monitoring of sleep in the artificial environment of the sleep laboratory may not accurately reflect real-world conditions at home and may overlook sleep problems. On the other hand, parents who are struggling with children with daytime behavior problems may be quicker to define even relatively minor sleep-related problems as severe in nature. They may be more likely to see the child's behavior in general in a negative light. Because of the night-to-night differences in sleep patterns in children with ADHD, parents may also be more likely to remember and report only the bad nights at home.

In any event, the question remains as to whether at least some children with ADHD, possibly a subgroup, have more intrinsic sleep problems (meaning they are basically born with it) that are not related to other factors, such as environmental issues, coexisting problems, or ADHD medications. Some ADHD experts have suggested that these children may have a higher arousal level that makes it difficult for them to "turn off" and settle down at bedtime. This may be why there is sometimes a surge in activity in the evening hours in these children followed by an abrupt "crash." Others have suggested that the production of the hormone melatonin, involved in the regulation of circadian rhythms, may be altered in at least some children with ADHD. This theory speculates that melatonin peaks later in some children with ADHD, resulting in a shift in bedtime and wake time to a later hour. This shift could, in turn, result in bedtime resistance if these children are required to go to bed earlier than the time their body clock demands.

On the other hand, some recent studies have suggested, counter to expectations, that some children with ADHD may actually be sleepier than other children. This raises the intriguing possibility that children with ADHD may be under- rather than *over*-stimulated. In this scenario, hyperactivity could, at least in some cases, actually be an adaptive behavior that is a response to feeling more sleepy during the day.

Finally, there may be links between the central nervous system centers that regulate sleep and those that regulate attention, arousal, and mood. Not only are common brain areas involved in sleep and attention, but some of the brain chemicals (neurotransmitters) that are known to be deficient or altered in ADHD are the same as those known to be involved in sleep and wake. This area in the brain is known as the prefrontal cortex and is located in the frontal lobe of the brain.

Common Sleep Problems in ADHD

Parents of children with ADHD often report that their child has had great difficulty in getting to sleep or has had difficulty sleeping since birth. They may complain that their child was unable or unwilling to take a nap, even when obviously exhausted. Many describe bedtime battles with a child who is overtired, yet fights sleep until he or she drops from exhaustion. This usually occurs long after the child's actual bedtime and way past the point when other family members are themselves ready to collapse. Other children with ADHD seem to want to fall asleep but are unable to do so, even when parents have worked hard to establish appropriate sleep routines. In still other children, the major complaint is difficulty falling back to sleep after waking during the night. Finally, some older children and adolescents, especially those with the more inattentive type of ADHD, having difficulty getting up in the morning. They also have problems staying awake and alert unless they are involved in a stimulating activity. Even when they are well rested, these children tend to become drowsy very quickly when they have to sit still for any length of time, such as when reading or when riding in a car.

Bedtime problems. For some children with ADHD and bedtime struggles, the problem is mostly one of parents having difficulties establishing bedtime rules and setting limits (see chapter 8). This is often a particular problem in children who have ADHD and are noncompliant and defiant during the day, as well.

BEDTIME PROBLEMS

- Do you find yourself dreading the battle that takes place every night when it's time for your child to go to bed?

- Does your child make a million demands for stories, drinks, hugs, etc. at bedtime?

- Does your child refuse to go to bed, even when he's obviously exhausted?

If you answered yes to any of these questions, see chapter 8.

Sleep associations. Other children with ADHD have problems with sleep associations; they never really learned to fall asleep by themselves, and often need help to go back to sleep during the night (see chapter 9).

SLEEP ASSOCIATIONS

• Does your child need you to be with him until he falls asleep?

• Does he wake up immediately if you try to leave the room?

• Does your child end up in your bed most nights?

If you answered yes to any of these questions, see chapter 9.

Anxiety issues. Children with ADHD and problems with anxiety may have more specific anxiety symptoms around sleep (see chapter 19).

ANXIETY ISSUES

• Does your child start to worry about going to bed once supper is over?

• Does she have difficulty being apart from you, even when you're just in another part of the house?

• Is your child so afraid of someone coming into the house at night that he can't fall asleep?

If you answered yes to any of these questions, see chapter 19.

Circadian rhythm problems. Especially with older children and teenagers, problems with falling asleep may be more related to a circadian rhythm problem in which the internal sleep-wake clock is shifted to a later time (see chapter 15).

CIRCADIAN RHYTHM PROBLEMS

• Does your teenager find it impossible to fall asleep at 10:00 PM on weekends but have no problem falling asleep at midnight on Friday night?

• During school vacation weeks, does your child just naturally fall asleep late and sleep until 10:00 AM or later?

• Does he feel more alert and ready to do his homework later in the evening?

If you answered yes to any of these questions, see chapter 15.

Poor sleep habits. Finally, for many children, it is a lack of good sleep habits or "sleep hygiene" that causes or worsens the sleep problems.

POOR SLEEP HABITS

• Does your child lack a regular bedtime and a "calm down" or relaxing routine at least a half-hour before lights-out?

• Does she drink beverages with caffeine late in the day?

• Is your child's bedtime and wake-up time much later on weekends than school days?

If you answered yes to any of these questions, see chapter 6.

Sleep Solutions

The most effective treatments for sleep problems for children with ADHD are those that directly address the cause(s) of the problem in that particular child. So the first step is to determine, as best as possible, which of the possible causes discussed above are most likely responsible for your child's sleep problems. This process includes looking for (and then treating) sleep problems like obstructive sleep apnea or inadequate sleep that might be causing or worsening the ADHD symptoms.

- **Don't assume your child with ADHD doesn't need much sleep.** Many children with ADHD, just like other children and teens, don't regularly get the sleep they need.
- **Check the drugs.** Some children's sleep problems are related to their ADHD medication. This can be a direct medication effect or a rebound effect as the medication is wearing off. The best indications are (1) if the sleep problem started at the same time medication was started, and (2) if your child falls asleep much more easily on those days when his medication was skipped or forgotten. If so, try changing the timing, the dose, or the type of medication. Some children may even benefit from a small dose of a short-acting ADHD medication near bedtime to reduce hyperactivity. There are also some medications used for ADHD, such as antidepressants and Strattera, that are not stimulants and seem to cause fewer sleep problems. In addition, these medications are effective in controlling ADHD symptoms for twenty-four hours a day, so evening ADHD behaviors may be decreased and bedtime is easier.
- **Treat other behavioral and psychiatric problems.** If your child's sleep problems seem mostly related to other problems, counseling and sometimes medication for these issues can be helpful.
- **Use what works.** Children with ADHD who also have bedtime problems or wake up at night generally respond well to the same strategies used in other children for these problems (see chapters 8 and 9).
- **Offer a reward.** Sticker charts and other reward systems can be very helpful. Because children with ADHD tend to become rapidly bored, you may need to be a bit more creative and frequently change the rewards in order to avoid "sticker burnout."
- **Shift bedtime.** Children who are night owls may do well with temporarily setting a later bedtime—that is, one that's closer to your child's natural fall-asleep time. Most parents of children with ADHD who already feel that the bedtime hour is a disaster are

horrified by the suggestion that they keep their child up even longer. However, this strategy actually has the effect of reducing a lot of the bedtime stress, because you are no longer fighting with your child about going to bed. And by the time the later bedtime does roll around, your child is much more likely to be ready to fall asleep. Once your child is falling asleep more easily, slowly move his bedtime earlier by fifteen to thirty minutes every few days. Be sure to keep your child's wake time the same.

- **Keep good sleep habits.** Make sure that poor habits are not contributing to your child's sleep problems. These include things like the sleeping environment (cooler temperature, low noise and light level), a regular sleep-wake schedule, and a consistent bedtime routine. Avoid habits that may make it more difficult for your child to fall asleep or stay asleep, such as exercising just before bed, going to bed hungry, eating a Big Mac just before bedtime, or drinking a caffeinated soft drink at 8:00 PM.
- **Stay calm.** Because children with ADHD may have more trouble settling down for bed, a relaxing bedtime routine that does not include stimulating activities like playing video games is especially important. Listening to a story, reading enjoyable (but not enjoyable enough to keep him awake) books, quietly talking, or listening to soothing music or relaxation tapes are more appropriate and more effective.
- **Use white noise.** If your child is particularly sensitive to environmental stimulation, a white noise machine, a noisy fan, or even the hum of a humidifier in the room may help muffle bothersome sounds. An eye mask can also screen out excessive light.
- **Ease into sleep.** Children with sensory integration problems may benefit from the use of occupational therapy techniques or using a body pillow at night. Talk with an occupational therapist for specific suggestions for your child.
- **Consider medication.** For some children with ADHD, the behavioral and other strategies described above don't seem to completely solve the sleep problems. In these children, particularly those in whom the sleep problems seem to worsen their daytime ADHD

symptoms, the use of a sleep medication at bedtime may be considered. However, it should be emphasized that there are currently no FDA-approved medications (either prescription or over-the-counter) for sleep problems in children or adolescents. And because there is very little information about the safety and efficacy of any sleep medication in children, these drugs should be used with a great deal of caution. Some of the medications that are prescribed for this purpose include clonidine, guanfacine (Tenex), prescription antihistamines, antidepressants, and a category of medication called *mood stabilizers*. Parents sometimes resort to using over-the-counter medications like Benadryl or herbal or "natural" preparations like chamomile or melatonin. Although generally thought to be safe, these medications have by and large not been tested specifically for sleep problems in children and may not be terribly effective. Finally, it's very important to inform your child's doctor if you are using any nonprescription medications or products to help your child sleep, as these could interfere with other medications that are being prescribed for ADHD. In all cases, medication should be combined with behavioral treatment and good sleep habits.

18

Sleepy Teens and the High Cost of Sleep Deprivation: What Parents and Schools Can Do

"I have a horrible time getting my sixteen-year-old daughter, Lindsey, up to go to school in the morning. I have to call up to her at least half a dozen times, and even then I usually end up physically dragging her out of bed. And she's always in a terrible mood in the morning, yelling at me and her brother and sister. But when I try to make her go to bed earlier at night, she tells me she has too much homework and she isn't tired anyway. I know this is affecting the whole family, but I don't know what to do."

Sound familiar? Any parent of a teenager knows this drill; the late nights up studying or on the Internet (well past the time that parents have gone to bed), the screaming matches the next morning, and the last-minute mad rush out the door to get to school on time. What a way to start the day! But this common scenario is played out every day in households across the United States, just like yours. And most parents (and teenagers) are no happier about the situation than you are.

So, given the obvious stress on everyone, why does it have to be this way? It would seem simple enough to just turn off the television and the computer, unplug the phone, and turn off the lights at 10:00 PM. But most parents of teens know it's a lot more complicated than that. Part of what you as a parent are up against is pure and simple biology. Some piece of it is also the very appropriate desire of teenagers to socialize and hang out with their friends. Another part is adolescents' increasing need for independence. Then there is the very real problem of all the other demands on a teenager's time, leaving less and less time available for sleep. Even if you could persuade your teen to stop instant messaging and go to bed at a decent hour, teachers still expect homework to be finished, the coach says the only time the hockey team can practice is from 8:00 to 9:00 PM, band practice is mandatory the week before the big concert, and that community service project has to be fit in somewhere. It just seems like there are too many priorities and not enough hours in the day.

Lots of parents caught in this situation get to the point where they give up trying to make their teenager get enough sleep, even though they can plainly see the consequences. Maybe they think that sleeping until noon on Saturday is enough to get caught up on sleep lost during the week. Or maybe they think that teenagers can get by on less sleep than the rest of us. Perhaps they've heard the argument that teens who can't get up for school in the morning are lazy and unmotivated. Or, most likely, they're not much better than their teenager about getting enough sleep themselves.

There is probably more controversy, lack of information, and misinformation about adolescents and sleep than about almost any other topic in sleep. In this chapter we explore the many causes and important consequences of sleep deprivation in teenagers, including the hidden toll on learning and academic success, and on the physical and mental health of adolescents. We also take a look at simpler and more complex possible solutions to this problem, and at some of the creative ways in which parents and schools in communities like yours have successfully approached it.

Sleep Changes in Adolescents: The Truth

Given all the physical and emotional upheaval that takes place in adolescence, it's not surprising that equally dramatic changes in sleep occur as well. And much like the other changes in adolescence, sleep patterns in teens represent a combination of biological, social, and psychological influences. Although researchers first began to notice and study these changing sleep patterns around the turn of the last century, it wasn't until the early 1990s that the work of Dr. Mary Carskadon and other sleep researchers substantially advanced our knowledge about how and why these changes occur. Although there is much that we don't yet fully understand, what we do know about normal sleep in teenagers helps us to make sense of their behavior and to find ways to encourage healthy sleep.

This is some of what the research shows about *how* teens sleep:

- **The body's sleep need does not really change in the teenage years.** Teenagers need almost as much sleep as preteens, about nine to ten hours per night. There may be a little individual variation in sleep needs (some need a little more, some need a little less), but studies have clearly shown that to function well, most teenagers need to sleep at least nine hours a night.
- **However, not surprisingly, most teenagers don't get nearly as much sleep as they need.** There have now been lots of studies performed in many countries and across many decades looking at the sleep habits of older children and adolescents. They all show the same thing: the vast majority of teens don't get anywhere near that magic number of nine to ten hours of sleep a night. In fact, on average, they get closer to seven hours. And the older your teenager, the less sleep she is likely to get. Recent studies have also shown that even younger adolescents and preteens are falling far short of their body's sleep requirements.
- **In comparison to school-aged children, teens have quite different sleep patterns.** First of all, they tend to have much later bedtimes and much earlier wake times. In addition, although children and preadolescents usually have approximately the same bedtime and wake-up time from one day to the next, teens typically go to bed much later and sleep much later on weekends than on school days. Finally, while children tend to sleep about the same length of time on school days as they do on non–school days, most adolescents sleep more (catch up on sleep) on weekends than they usually do during the week.

Recent research has also shown us a lot about why teens don't get the sleep they need:

- **They can't fight biology.** During puberty, important changes occur in the way that the body's circadian system works. Circadian rhythms act as the body's timekeeper, particularly when it comes to determining when we sleep and when we are awake. For example, some people are "night owls," meaning they prefer to go to bed and get up relatively later. Others are more like "morning larks" (these are the folks who leap out of bed at 6:00 AM, bright-eyed and bushy-tailed). This preference for when we sleep is biologically based, which means it is both built into our genetic makeup and controlled by specialized centers in our brain. Dr. Carskadon and her colleagues were the first to show that all teenagers have a normal shift in their circadian rhythms to a later bedtime and wake-up time (on average, two hours later) that happens around the years of puberty. This means that your fifteen-year-old simply can't fall asleep at the same time as her twelve-year-old brother. Her body is also telling her to sleep later in the morning. And if she was a night owl to begin with, her natural fall-asleep time and wake-up time shifted even later as she started to go through puberty.

- **They have competing priorities.** Like everyone else, teenagers have a million competing priorities for sleep time and a million and one reasons why they want to ("have to") stay up until all hours. Some of the reasons are good ones (homework, extracurricular activities), some not so good (watching television, playing computer games), and some are okay up to a point (socializing with friends, working at after-school jobs). But the bottom line is, sleep always seems to be the one activity that gets the short end of the stick.

- **They have to go to school.** And for many teenagers, school starts early. Many school districts in the United States currently use a three- or four-tier schedule, in which high schools start first in the morning, followed by middle (or junior high) schools, and then elementary schools. In 1996–1997, a study of forty high schools throughout the United States showed that almost half started at 7:30 AM or earlier. More recently, in 2001–2002, a survey of fifty high schools found that 35 percent started earlier than 7:30 AM, and only 16 percent started classes between the more reasonable hours of 8:15 and 8:55 AM.

- **They pay to play.** Another major influence on sleep patterns of high-school students in the United States is the number of hours they spend working at after-school jobs to pay for things like clothes, gas, and entertainment. In one recent study, nearly 60 percent of high-school students reported that they held part-time jobs, and almost 30 percent indicated that they worked twenty hours or more a week. Those students who work more than twenty hours per week at an after-school job go to bed later and sleep less. They also have a harder time getting up, are more likely to fall asleep in class, and report struggling to stay awake while driving, reading, studying, or doing homework. As a result, these teenagers are also more likely to use stimulants like caffeine and tobacco, as well as stimulant drugs, to stay awake.

- **They're on their own.** Parents have often stopped setting and supervising bedtime by the time their teenager reaches high school. Only about 5 percent of ninth through twelfth-graders have their school-night bedtime set by their parents, and more than 75 percent of them go to bed only when homework, television viewing, or socializing is done for the day, or whenever they feel sleepy (whichever come first). On the other hand, in contrast to younger children who usually wake up by themselves, more than 85 percent of high-school students depend on an alarm or their parents to wake them up in the morning on school days. So the influence of parents shifts away from setting bedtimes during childhood to becoming more involved with the morning wake-up call in the teenage years.

- **They have sleep disorders, too.** Finally, there are teenagers who don't get the sleep they need as a result of having a sleep disorder. For example, adolescents with obstructive sleep apnea (see chapter 13), for which overweight and obese teens may be particularly at risk, are often sleepy and fatigued during the day. Delayed sleep phase syndrome (see chapter 15), another common sleep disorder in adolescents, causes problems with falling asleep at a normal bedtime. Possible symptoms of sleep disorders in sleepy teens such as loud nightly snoring, extremely restless sleep, or kicking movements during the night, should definitely be brought to the attention of your child's doctor. However, these cases are the exception rather than the rule.

THE BOTTOM LINE

Just not getting enough sleep, pure and simple, accounts for 90 percent of daytime sleepiness in adolescents.

Sleep Changes in Adolescents: The Consequences

So teenagers need sleep; don't we all? None of us in the twenty-four-hour-supermarket, all-night-cable-television, gotta-stay-ahead-of-the-next-guy-seven-days-a-week modern world we live in get enough sleep either. We do okay, don't we? We're at the top of our game, just like Donald Trump (who boasts about getting only four hours of sleep a night), aren't we? Maybe not. Maybe we really do need those three cups of coffee in the morning just to get ourselves going. Or maybe we're just so exhausted all the time, we no longer notice how tired we are.

Leaving aside for a minute the fact that you may not be the world's best role model for sleep, as a parent of a teenager it is especially important to fully understand the very real price that many teens pay for not getting enough sleep. And the costs are pretty steep, considering that they can include depression, poor grades, and an increase in accidental injuries, including car accidents, just to mention a few. Moreover, teenagers are likely to be at greater risk than adults for almost any consequence of inadequate sleep that you can name. They have fewer coping skills to deal with it, and their judgment about how compromised they are is often quite poor.

So what are the costs? Well, no surprise, the most common effect of sleep deprivation is sleepiness. Sounds like a no-brainer, right? What might not be so obvious is the fact that human beings, in general, are terrible judges of both how sleepy we are and how much the sleepiness affects us. And the sleepier you are, the less likely you are to recognize it (and thus to do something about it!). So asking a teenager if not getting enough sleep is a problem for him is kind of like asking if he thinks his hair is too long; it's all in the eye of the beholder (and it's just fine, thanks). And if that weren't enough, people who are really sleep deprived can actually fall asleep for several seconds (microsleeps) *without realizing they are asleep*. Think about that the next time your teenager is driving home late at night.

Then there is the large amount of research that supports what every parent of a sleep-deprived teenager knows: that there is a relationship between an adolescent not getting enough sleep and changes in mood. These include less positive moods, more negative emotional responses, and more mood swings. At one end of the spectrum, this explains the sullen teenager riding to school with you in the morning. At the other end, it provides a potential link between the parallel decrease in sleep time and increase in depression in adolescents that we've seen over the past few decades. Sleep problems are clearly more common in teenagers who have been diagnosed with clinical depression and vice versa. Furthermore, improvements in sleep often result in improvements in the depression symptoms as well.

In addition, sleep deprivation is particularly likely to affect people's ability to think and make decisions when they are emotionally stressed ("grace under pressure"). This becomes pretty important when you consider how much of an adolescent's life revolves around doing what they need to do while dealing with new and often intense emotions. Sleep deprivation makes doing so even more difficult. All of this can lead to a downward spiral of late nights and irregular sleep schedules, resulting in sleep deprivation, which affects mood and creates more stress. Increased stress causes more difficulties with sleep, resulting in yet more mood problems, and more difficulty functioning at home, at school, and with friends. And so on and so on.

High-school students are also often struggling with enormous academic demands and pressures. Not only does the workload in high school increase dramatically, but the difficulty of the material and the need for more organization and time management skills increase as well. Students are expected to multitask, prioritize, sort through tons of information efficiently and accurately, and think creatively. Unfortunately, these are the very skills that research shows are most compromised by loss of sleep. Not to mention the higher rates of tardiness, the increased absenteeism, and the higher dropout rates that have been linked to inadequate sleep in high-school students. Attitudes and motivation may suffer as well. Studies show that students who are well rested are more likely to be receptive to teachers, to have a more positive self-image, and to report being more motivated to do their best in school than their sleepier peers.

Getting by on less than enough sleep becomes less of an option the more academically successful your teenager aspires to be. In fact, contrary to what you might think, teenagers who get less sleep (even if they are staying up late to study) and have less regular sleep schedules have a lower level of academic achievement. The opposite is also true. A and B students report going to bed earlier and getting more sleep than students with poorer grades. Looking beyond high school, sleep habits are more important in predicting grade point averages in first-year college students than eating habits, mood, stress, time management, and social support. In addition, students who sleep at least nine hours a night have better grades than those who sleep six hours or less.

Other high-risk behaviors have been found more frequently in sleep-deprived teens as well. These include higher rates of alcohol and drug use and higher rates of cigarette smoking, as well as abuse of nonprescription stimulants like caffeine and prescription drugs like Ritalin. In some cases, teens may be using the stimulant effects of one substance (like nicotine) to keep themselves awake during the day, while at the same time they are taking advantage of the drowsiness effect of another substance (alcohol, marijuana) to counteract these stimulants and help them fall asleep at night. Add in the effects of alcohol or drugs in a given situation (like driving home from a party) in which a teenager's judgment, motor skills, and ability to react may already be compromised by sleep loss, and the result could be deadly.

In fact, those who are most likely to be involved in fall-asleep crashes are young people (especially young men) between the ages of sixteen and twenty-nine. Other risk factors include being an inexperienced driver and taking more risks on the road, both of which certainly apply to most teenagers. Across drivers of all age, about 60 percent report having driven while sleepy in the past year, and over one-third have fallen asleep at the wheel. And to think that the numbers are much higher for teenagers!

Drowsy-driving crashes involving teenagers often take place during the very early morning hours (unlike drowsy-driving accidents in the elderly, which typically occur in the mid-afternoon hours). The drivers are usually alone, and when the car veers off the road, the result is often fatal, because the driver is asleep and therefore makes little effort to avoid the crash. *It takes only a four-second microsleep to result in a crash.* Most people don't realize at that point that they've even been asleep. Both how much you slept the night(s) before and how long you've been awake play an important role in causing these types of accidents. Compared to sleeping eight or more hours each night, sleeping six to seven hours is associated with almost twice the risk for having a fall-asleep crash. Sleeping less than five hours per night more than quadruples the risk. Forty percent of drivers involved in a drowsy-driving crash in one study had been awake for fifteen or more hours before the accident, and nearly 20 percent had been awake for more than twenty hours.

The risk of drowsy-driving crashes in adolescents may be even higher than these statistics suggest. Police officers and emergency workers aren't always trained to ask about sleep deprivation as a possible cause of a crash. In addition, because there is nothing like a Breathalyzer test or test for blood alcohol level to measure sleepiness, many of these accidents may be missed or blamed on drugs or alcohol. *And remember, even a very small amount of alcohol combined with sleep deprivation has the same effect as drinking much more.* Driving while drowsy is also very common in this age group. In one study, two-thirds of college students admitted to driving while sleep-impaired. However, most of these students also downplayed the risks of this behavior, even when they knew someone who had been involved in a drowsy-driving accident.

So What's a Parent (or a School System) to Do?

Hopefully, you are now convinced that making sure your teenager gets enough sleep ranks right up there with making sure he eats right, gets regular exercise, wears his seatbelt, and never takes up smoking. It should. But as you can see, the odds are stacked against you. Your opponents in this struggle for shut-eye are many (the Internet, cable TV, cell phones, teachers, girl/boyfriends, coaches, college admission officers) and powerful (society in general, your teenager himself). As if that weren't bad enough, your kids are likely to get more health education in school about what number SPF sunscreen to use than they are about what they spend a third of their lives doing.

But the good news is that you've taken the first (and most important) step by reading this book. And more good news is that there are a lot of parents just like you who are struggling with these problems and trying just as hard as you are to find solutions. There are also a lot more resources available now for parents, schools, and health care professionals about adolescent sleep than there were even two or three years ago. And perhaps best of all, there are now a growing number of school systems in the United States that have heard the wake-up call about school start times, and even some who have taken on the responsibility of educating their students about the importance of sleep.

The Campaign at Home. Most of what parents can do, besides being aware of the problem to begin with and recognizing the sometimes-subtle signs of sleep deprivation in their teenagers, is to provide the infrastructure for good sleep to happen. This means creating a sleep-friendly home environment (keep televisions and computers out of the bedroom), making sleep a lifestyle priority for the whole family (avoid scheduling late-night activities, help your teenager to manage his time more efficiently), and, yes, acting as a "good sleep citizen" yourself (leave the party early, forgo Letterman once in a while). It also means sometimes acting like the ogre your kids accuse you of already being and setting limits. Limits on the amount of TV they watch, the number of caffeinated beverages they drink, the hours during which they are allowed to call their friends, the number of extracurricular activities they participate in, and the hours they work at after-school jobs. And setting there's-no-arguing-with-this-one limits on your teenager driving without getting enough sleep, or riding in a car with a sleep-deprived driver (let's face it, this is the best carrot and stick you have). The third piece, and probably the most difficult one, involves being a sleep advocate for your teen by occasionally challenging the status quo of teachers, coaches, and school administrators, who sometimes place inappropriate and unreasonable roadblocks in the way of adequate sleep.

Of course, all of this would have been a lot easier if you had started it while your child could still stand being in the same room with you ("you're not actually going to wear that in front of my friends, are you?"). And before eye rolling became her principal means of communication. So, as with anything else involving adolescents, you have to make it seem like it was her idea. Gently point out how much happier she seems (and better she looks) when she's gotten a good night's sleep for a few days in a row. Casually leave magazine articles around about the effects of inadequate sleep on whatever-she-cares-about (academic achievement, weight gain, driving skills). Mention in passing that perhaps the fact that the soccer coach always reminds the team to get enough sleep on the night before the big game is an indication that sleep is an important part of her athletic success (and she owes it to the team). Carefully suggest that turning on a bright light in her room in the morning is actually not a form of child abuse, but rather your well-meaning (and scientifically based) attempt to help her to wake up (by shutting down her body's production of melatonin, the "sleep hormone"). It's worth a try, and, who knows, it could work.

The Campaign at School. Obviously another important partner in your campaign for healthy sleep is the school in which your teenager spends a good part of his waking (and not so awake) hours. What can schools do?

- Give a clear message to students that sleep is not optional or just a luxury; it's as important as eating and breathing.
- Include sleep as a part of student health education and biology classes. There is an excellent curriculum for students in grades nine through twelve on sleep, sleep disorders, and circadian biology that is available through the National Center for Sleep Disorders Research Web site (www.nhlbi.nih.gov/about/ncsdr).
- Educate all school personnel—teachers, nurses, coaches, administrators, and school counselors—about the importance of sleep for adolescents.
- Include education about drowsy driving in all driver education classes (again, excellent resources may be found at www.nhlbi. nih.gov/about/ncsdr and www.drowsydriving.org). Schools need to help get the message across that drowsy driving is as dangerous —and as avoidable—as drunk driving. Students should be educated about how to avoid driving while drowsy and strongly encouraged to find safe alternatives to driving when they're feeling

tired, such as assigning someone to be a designated (alert) driver, arranging to get a ride home, or staying at a friend's house overnight.

• Help students manage their schedules so that they have time for adequate sleep. Brainstorm techniques for building sleep into their busy schedules.

DRIVE ALERT . . . ARRIVE ALIVE!

• Get enough sleep before a car trip, especially a long one.
• Avoid driving between 2:00 AM and 6:00 AM (peak sleepiness time).
• Schedule regular driving breaks—every 100 miles or two hours.
• Take along a passenger who can help you stay alert and can let you know if you are getting sleepy.
• Don't mix driving and sedating medications (antihistamines, antidepressants, etc.).
• Never mix alcohol and drowsy driving.

And, finally, if you are now brave enough to take on the school system in your community about school start times, here's some ammunition. The National Sleep Foundation (www.sleepfoundation.org) is also an excellent resource for information on changing high-school start times.

• Studies show that students who start school at 7:30 AM or earlier get less sleep on school nights. For example, in one large high school that started at 7:20 AM, only 62 percent of ninth-graders and fewer than half of tenth-graders got an average of even seven hours of sleep on school nights. In another study of younger adolescents (ages ten to twelve), children with early start times (7:10 AM) slept about twenty-five minutes less than did children who started school at 8:00 AM.
• Studies also show that these students have more school problems. One study that compared adolescents who started school at 7:15 AM or earlier with those who started at 8:00 AM found that the earlier risers complained more of daytime fatigue and sleepiness throughout

the school day, had a greater tendency to doze off in class, and had more attention and concentration difficulties in school.

- Here is perhaps the most convincing argument to date. Beginning with the 1997–1998 school year, Minneapolis Public Schools were smart enough to change their high-school start time from 7:15 AM to 8:40 AM. They also were smart enough to study the outcomes (grades, school attendance, sleep habits) of this decision in great detail. Although this is an ongoing project, which will give us lots of information in the coming years, what they know so far is this:
  - Daily attendance rates improved.
  - The percentage of high-school students who stayed in school increased, and the dropout rate decreased.
  - There was no change in the students' average school-night bedtimes. However, because they were able to sleep later in the morning, students reported that they got *one hour more sleep per night* (or five hours more per week) on school nights than students in high schools with an earlier start. This clearly challenges the popular argument against delaying school start times that says students will just stay up later and thus not get any more sleep.
  - Other improvements that students report related to this change in school start times include getting better grades, feeling less depressed, and even being more likely to eat breakfast! Teachers also report that students are more alert during their first two classes in particular, are less likely to fall asleep, and have fewer behavior problems overall.

Despite all the obvious positives, there are clearly some real challenges involved for school systems that are considering delaying school start times. Bus transportation, the potential effect on school schedules at other levels (elementary, middle school), the scheduling of athletic programs and extracurricular activities, and food services schedules are just some of the issues that need to be looked at carefully. School buildings may also be used for other purposes, such as community groups and day care, during the mid- to late-afternoon hours. In some communities the greatest amount of opposition to changing the high-school start time has come not from the school administration. Parents who rely on older siblings to provide after-school child care for their younger brothers and sisters may be against the change. And students themselves are often reluctant to give up the extra hours spent at after-school jobs. Don't let all of this discourage you. There are now many schools across the country that have met these challenges and have successfully managed to change the system for the better. Yours can, too. But you'll need to do your homework in helping to educate your school and your community about the very real benefits of making the change, as well as the very real risks of failing to do so.

19

Sleep Problems in Children with Medical, Emotional, and Developmental Special Needs

Augustin is seven years old and was diagnosed with autism when he was three. He falls asleep with little problem at 8.30 at night, but invariably is awake by 3:00 in the morning. Most nights, he doesn't fall back to sleep until 5:00 AM. Although there are some nights when he just stays up for the day.

Stephanie is sixteen and was recently diagnosed with juvenile rheumatoid arthritis. The pain makes it hard for her to sleep at night, and then she feels worse the next day because she's exhausted. It's a vicious cycle.

Children and adolescents with chronic medical conditions (such as asthma), behavioral/emotional disorders (such as ADHD or depression), or developmental disorders (such as autism or Down syndrome) are more likely to have sleep problems than other children. These sleep problems are often the same ones that affect other kids, such as obstructive sleep apnea and nightmares; however, they may also be related to the underlying problem. For example, children with painful medical conditions like juvenile rheumatoid arthritis (JRA) may have less restful sleep because of joint pain. Children with asthma often wheeze more during the night, which disrupts their sleep. Asthma medications can also have negative effects on sleep. Children who are anxious or depressed may have more difficulty falling asleep and wake more at night. In addition, many medications used for depression and anxiety can cause sleep problems. Autistic children and children with severe developmental delays often have a great deal of difficulty settling at night. They may also have very irregular sleep patterns, which may be partly related to the way that their brains are wired.

A lot of these children are also more vulnerable to the toll that sleep problems can take on physical and mental health. In other words, having a sleep problem in addition to another condition can make the condition worse. Take again the example of a child with juvenile rheumatoid arthritis—pain at night results in poor sleep, poor sleep causes daytime tiredness, and daytime tiredness makes the pain seem worse. And so on. Not getting enough sleep can also have very negative effects on the immune system and the body's ability to respond to stress, which can also clearly complicate medical problems. Because one of the main consequences of not getting enough sleep is moodiness and irritability, adolescents who are already depressed or anxious may become that much more depressed or anxious if they are not sleeping well or not sleeping enough. Children with learning and attention problems often do worse with less sleep. (For more about ADHD and sleep, see chapter 17).

In addition, children (and their exhausted parents), when they are poorly rested and overtired, have more limited coping skills. They are less able to deal with their illness or problem, because sleep deprivation results in lower frustration tolerance and less control of emotions. For the same reason, even their compliance with treatment (taking medication, doing physical therapy, attending counseling sessions) can be negatively affected. Looking at the glass as half-full, however, when you improve sleep in these kids, you often make the asthma, depression, or attention problems better as well.

Sleep problems in children with other issues can also have a huge impact on the family. Parents who are already stressed from worrying about their child, and exhausted from all the many caretaking responsibilities that they have, are even more likely to suffer when their child is not getting enough sleep or is up at night. For some of these families, the added exhaustion of sleepless nights becomes the straw that broke the camel's back. At times, parents can also unknowingly contribute to sleep problems. For example, sometimes parents are so concerned about their child that they don't always discipline when they should. Or they may be so frazzled and fried that setting limits at bedtime or dealing with night wakings is the last thing they want to do. But be forewarned that this situation can be a set-up for behavioral sleep problems. Short-term fixes (letting your child come into bed with you, for example) can lead to long-term worsening of the sleep problem.

The key here, as has been emphasized throughout this book, is that parents need to be aware of the potential for sleep problems, especially in children with medical or emotional or developmental issues. They need to recognize the link between sleep problems and daytime functioning in these children. And they need to bring any sleep issues to the attention of their child's doctor (or therapist or counselor). A few of the most common issues are covered in this chapter.

Medications

Many of the medications that are used for a variety of medical and psychiatric conditions can lead to sleep problems or make them worse. For example, pain medications, even though they may improve sleep by reducing pain at night, may have side effects (such as stomach upset) that can make sleep worse. Some medications seem to directly affect sleep, causing difficulty falling asleep or restless sleep. Others actually affect sleep stages (see chapter 2). In this case, withdrawal from the drug may be more of a problem. For example, medications (like some antidepressants) that reduce the amount of REM sleep or "dream sleep" can result in what is called *REM rebound* (increased REM sleep) when the medication is stopped. And this increase in REM sleep can lead to a temporary increase in dreaming, more vivid dreams, and even nightmares.

Many of the medications used to treat children with medical problems can also make your child sleepy during the day. The sleepiness can then interfere with daytime functioning and also with nighttime sleep. For example, sleeping during the day can make it more difficult to fall asleep that night. Although, in theory, almost any medication can cause almost any side effect on any given day, the following is a list of some medications that are more likely to cause sleep problems. If in doubt, ask your child's doctor about whether a particular medication that your child is taking might affect your child's sleep.

COMMON MEDICATIONS THAT CAN INTERFERE WITH SLEEP

Pain medications
  Ibuprofen, codeine
Asthma medications
  Especially theophylline, prednisone
Allergy and cold medications
  Antihistamines are more likely to cause sleepiness
  Decongestants are more likely to cause disrupted sleep
Seizure medications
  Often cause sleepiness
Antidepressants
  Some cause difficulty falling sleep and sleep disruption
  Others cause sleepiness
Stimulants
  Ritalin/Concerta, Adderall/Dexedrine, caffeine, nicotine

It's also important to remember that not all children react in the same way to a particular medication. So what knocks Evan out in a heartbeat (such as a cough suppressant with codeine) may not faze Grace in the least. Some kids may even have what's known as a "paradoxical" or opposite reaction to a medication. Instead of Benadryl putting them right to sleep, it (literally) creates a wild monster.

Sometimes your child's doctor can switch to a different medication. For example, many of the newer medications for asthma have very little effect on sleep when compared to some of the older ones like theophylline (although some, like Singulair, can cause insomnia in some people). If being sleepy during the day is a side effect of a particular antihistamine (such as Claritin or Zyrtec), many children with allergies can successfully switch to a "newer-generation" antihistamine that does not cause drowsiness. Some antidepressants (particularly the type known as SSRIs, such as Prozac) are more likely to result in difficulties falling and staying asleep. So a more sedating antidepressant (such as Remeron or Celexa) may be helpful if sleep problems are part of the depression. Although in many cases it is not possible to switch medications if a sleep problem occurs, it's definitely worth raising the possibility with your child's doctor.

Hospitalization

Stephen was rushed to the hospital for an emergency appendectomy. He was in the hospital for a total of three days. He barely slept while he was there. There was too much noise, the nurses kept checking on him all night, and he was too anxious. His parents hoped that when he got home, he would sleep better. But once he got home, he insisted on one of his parents staying with him all night, and he woke up throughout the night to check that they were still there.

Hospitalization is very stressful for children and their families. Children, especially younger ones, may react to this stress by becoming clingier and more dependent on adults, especially on parents. They may temporarily slip back or regress to behaviors they had when they were much younger. On top of that, parents are often worried and distracted, regular home routines (including bedtime) are disrupted, and the hospital environment (the beeping noises, bright lights, constant interruptions) is not exactly conducive to a good night's sleep. One study found that children in a pediatric intensive care unit got, on average, less than five hours of sleep a night!

For all of these reasons, sleep problems are very common in children who are hospitalized. Obviously, there are limits on what a parent can do in this situation, but the following tips can help:

- **Bring sleep stuff from home.** If the hospital will allow it, it's very comforting to have one's own jammies, pillow, and stuffed bunny (even when you're sixteen) with you at bedtime.
- **Keep to home routines as much as possible.** This includes things like your child's regular bedtime, bedtime snack, bedtime routine, story, and song.
- **Bring pictures of family members.** Most hospitals these days allow parents to stay with their child overnight. But if you can't stay, have photos of you, your child's brothers and sisters, and the family dog on your child's bedside table. (Note: Surprisingly, some studies have found that a parent rooming-in and reminders of home may actually make for more sleep problems in some kids. Clearly this will vary with a child's personality and age. Use your own judgment, as you know your child best.)

- **Relax.** The use of relaxation and imagery techniques can be a godsend for the hospitalized or sick child. Try a relaxation CD at bedtime or one of those (fairly expensive) "soothing sound" generators from Brookstone or Sharper Image (a less expensive white noise generator from Radio Shack can work just as well for some kids). These techniques can help create the state of physical and mental relaxation needed for sleep, reduce noise, provide distraction, and can often help reduce pain.
- **No needles.** Unfortunately, blood draws, needle sticks, and IVs are often part of the hospital experience. You can help ease the pain of these and other painful or scary procedures by asking that your child's bed, if possible, be a safe "no needle" zone. That way, being in bed (especially when it's time to go to sleep) will not be associated in your child's imagination with getting hurt and feeling scared.
- **Expect some backsliding.** It's very normal for kids, when they are under stress and away from home, to temporarily slip back into old (comforting) behaviors that they had given up long before, like needing a parent to stay with them at bedtime. Temporary difficulties in falling or staying asleep are very common (and normal) reactions to stress (in adults as well as kids!).
- **Get back to normal as quickly as possible.** Once the dust has settled and everyone is back home and back to normal, regular bedtime rules and routines should be put back in place as well. A very common mistake that parents make, once the crisis has passed, is to continue to allow their child to sleep in bed with them, go to bed later than usual, have a television set in the bedroom, or indulge in other bad habits. On face value, this impulse is very understandable and sounds like what any caring parent would do. But the reality is that what started out as a small temporary sleep problem can very quickly become a big bad habit (and much harder to get rid of!). So hang tough and do the right thing.

Allergies and Asthma

Jenna was diagnosed with asthma when she was three. Her asthma is much worse during the winter, because she usually gets lots of colds. She often wakes up at night coughing and then has a hard time falling back to sleep.

Danny has terrible eczema and is itchy all night. His parents slather him with lotion at bedtime, but he is still up several times at night scratching.

Seasonal or year-round allergies are common in kids and can cause sleep problems or make them worse. An allergy-related runny or stuffy nose, scratchy throat, or chronic cough (which is often made worse at night by a post-nasal drip down the back of the throat) often makes for an uncomfortable night. Children with skin allergies and eczema are particularly likely to have disrupted sleep as a result of all the itching and scratching that goes on at night. Allergies are also often associated with frequent sinus infections and with asthma, both of which may make sleep even worse. Nearly 60 percent of kids with asthma have sleep problems. Asthma symptoms in particular are often worse at night, and in some children occur mainly at night ("nocturnal asthma"). Asthma also increases the risk for obstructive sleep apnea (see chapter 13).

Adequate nighttime control of symptoms, such as wheezing, coughing, and itching, with medications that do not further disrupt sleep is key. In addition, many children with allergies (and asthma) do much better at night when allergens in the bedroom are controlled as much as possible. Use protective mattress and pillow covers and hypoallergenic pajamas. Run an air filter, dust and vacuum frequently, and remove stuffed animals from the bed. And, finally, much to your child's dismay, keep Rover and Puff-Puff out of the bedroom. Be sure to discuss both your child's daytime and nighttime symptoms with your child's doctor to make sure your child's asthma and allergies are well controlled through the entire day and night.

Developmental Issues

Timothy is nine years old and has Down syndrome. He snores incredibly loudly at night and often falls asleep in school.

Juan is eleven years old and is developmentally delayed. He was born prematurely at thirty weeks and has major cognitive delays. His developmental age is about that of a three-year-old. He falls asleep with one of his parents and wakes up several times a night. He almost always ends up in his parents' bed. He's gotten so big that either his father or mother ends up sleeping in the guest bedroom, because there just isn't enough room in the bed for all of them.

Children who have developmental delays or mental retardation, like autism, Fragile X syndrome, and Down syndrome, are particularly susceptible to sleep problems. About 70–80 percent of autistic children have sleep problems, and up to 70 percent of children with Down syndrome have obstructive sleep apnea. These sleep problems often take a terrible toll on families. However, sometimes parents are reluctant to bring them to the attention of their child's doctor, because they think that they are "just part of the condition" and nothing can be done.

Fortunately, they are wrong. Most sleep problems in children with developmental delays can be successfully treated, although not always eliminated. It usually takes a combination of behavioral strategies and sometimes medication. Furthermore, many of these sleep problems respond well to the same behavioral management techniques that work for other children.

In general, it is just as important to maintain good sleep practices (see chapter 6) for special-needs children as it is for typically developing children. Parents are often surprised by how small changes in sleep habits, such as set bedtimes and having their child fall asleep independently, can make a world of difference. The only real difference is that it often takes much longer before positive changes are seen. Whereas a typically developing child may start sleeping through the night in a week or two, it may take a month or two with a developmentally delayed child. Therefore, don't get discouraged if you don't see changes right away. You have to stick with it.

Unfortunately, a complete discussion of dealing with sleep issues in these special-needs children is impossible to cover here. Therefore, for more detailed information in dealing with sleep problems in special-needs children, see the excellent resources listed in appendix B.

Mood and Anxiety Disorders

Dana, who is fourteen, has been depressed for about a year. Since she started taking an antidepressant and seeing a therapist, she has gotten much better. Her mood has improved and she is starting to get back to spending time with her friends and getting involved at school. However, she still finds that it is often hard to fall asleep at night and many nights she wakes up at 4:00 or 5:00 AM and can't get back to sleep. After a night of little sleep, she can feel herself slipping back into the depression.

As has been stated many times in this book, there is clearly a two-way relationship between sleep and mood/behavior. That is, each affects the other. Not getting enough sleep leads to moodiness, unclear thinking, poor attention span, and behavior problems. On the flip side, up to 90 percent of children and adolescents diagnosed with depression and anxiety disorders experience sleep disturbances. In addition, other behaviors associated with anxiety and depression in adolescents, such as alcohol use, smoking, and drug abuse, may make sleep problems even more likely. Difficulties in falling and staying sleep are also often related to acute or chronic anxiety.

Because sleep disturbances and mood/anxiety disorders often go together, the most effective treatment usually involves dealing with both concerns at the same time. At the very least, make sure the treatment chosen for the emotional condition doesn't make any sleep problems worse—for instance, using an antidepressant or anxiety medication that can have negative effects on sleep. When dealing with sleep problems in a child or adolescent with anxiety, it's important to distinguish between more temporary nighttime anxiety (nighttime fears) and sleep symptoms that are related to more severe and frequent daytime anxiety. What will help your child in each of these situations is likely to be quite different. For example, most of the recommendations provided in chapter 10 will work extremely well if the main problem is that your child is scared of the dark. However, if your child is also extremely anxious during the day, it is best to seek out counseling for her. A therapist will help you and your child develop the management strategies and coping skills needed before nighttime issues can be tackled. Children who have more serious anxiety often need much more intensive and longer-term treatment, and behavioral strategies may have to be introduced much more gradually.

20

Sleep Drugs: Should You Use Medication to Help Your Child Sleep?

Alicia's parents are at their wit's end. For the past year, Alicia has been waking up at night, up to five times each night. They are ready to call their pediatrician and ask for drugs to get her to sleep.

Anthony has cerebral palsy, and it takes him up to an hour to fall asleep at bedtime. He is also up several times a night. Most times he falls right back to sleep, but sometimes he is up for hours. It's impossible for his parents to tell what is wrong. Is he in pain? Is he uncomfortable? Or does he just want attention? Anthony's doctors have prescribed different medications in the hopes of helping him sleep better at night. They've had limited success.

The initial response (and second and even third) to the question "Should I give my child (should my teenager take) something to help her sleep?" is NO (no, no). There are lots of very good reasons not to, chief among them is that there are no prescription or over-the-counter medications that have been approved for use in the United States for children or adolescents who have difficulty falling asleep or staying asleep. Which basically means that the federal government agencies-that-be (such as the FDA) have concluded that we don't have enough information about either the benefits or the risks of any sleep medications in children to make them a safe bet. And the majority of the time, medication is not the best (or even the second or third best) treatment choice.

Nevertheless, medications are being used. In a study we conducted a few years ago of pediatricians from all over the country, more than 75 percent of the doctors reported that they had recommended an over-the-counter medication, and 50 percent said that they had prescribed a sleep medication at least once in the past six months. Now we don't know how many times that happened (it may have been only that one time), but this suggests that prescribing medication for sleep disorders is a fairly common practice. The study also did not tell us how many parents were giving their child an over-the-counter or herbal sleep medication without their doctor's knowledge. However, it is reasonable to conclude that parents are complaining about sleep problems to their pediatricians, and the pediatricians are responding to those complaints, at least in some percentage of cases, by suggesting medication for sleep. So on the one hand, we have what seems to be a real practical need (or at least the perception of one) for sleep medications for children. On the other hand, though, we have very little scientific information about how and when and what should be used, and whether or not it's safe.

If this sounds like a bit of a mixed-message, it is. We realize that there may be situations in which you as a parent might want to consider giving your child a medicine to get him to sleep. Some of those situations have to do with short-term sleep problems, such as an ear infection or traveling on an airplane. Other times it is because of a serious and much more chronic sleep problem, such as in children with autism. Another possible scenario is the anxious adolescent who requests something to help her fall asleep the night before the big exam. If you do not believe that medication for sleep is ever appropriate for a child (and remember, herbal or "natural" medications are drugs, too), we certainly respect your judgment as a parent and applaud your choice. However, if you do accept the idea that some medication might be appropriate for treating difficulties falling or staying asleep in some children at some point for some period of time, read on for the rules of the game.

Rule 1: Never give a sleep medication to your child without first consulting your doctor.

Even "harmless" over-the-counter medications that are commonly used to help kids sleep (Benadryl comes immediately to mind) can have side effects or can cause problems if they are mixed with other medications. Sometimes parents don't realize that the main ingredient in one medication they are giving their child (Benadryl = diphenhydramine) is the same as one of the ingredients in another medication they are giving at the same time (over-the-counter medications for cold or allergy symptoms frequently also contain diphenhydramine). *This mixing of medications can result in an overdose!*

Herbal or "natural" sleep medications in pill form and in things like tea (chamomile, kava-kava, valerian) are generally believed to be safe for children in appropriate amounts. However, again, we don't really have much data on their safety. You may remember, a number of years ago, the herbal sleep product tryptophan (same as the nap-inducing ingredient in your Thanksgiving Day turkey) was withdrawn from the market, because it was linked to a serious blood disorder. Herbal medications can also have interactions with other drugs your child may be taking. So talk with your doctor first!

Rule 2: Never give a sleep medication without making sure there is no other reason for the sleep problem.
This could also easily be rule 1. Insomnia, or difficulty falling asleep or staying asleep, is a symptom and not a diagnosis. This means that there could be dozens of potential causes for the same set of symptoms that need to be checked out. For example, difficulty falling asleep could be the result of a too-early bedtime, delayed sleep phase syndrome, oppositional behavior, restless legs syndrome, or a decongestant medication being taken for allergies. Clearly, the treatment for each of these is quite different. And the treatment for sleep problems, in order to be successful, has to match the cause.

Rule 3: Sleep medication should always be combined with behavioral treatment.
Study after study in both adults and children with insomnia have shown that, in the long run, the behavior changes, not the medication, make the difference in the successful treatment of sleep problems. Medication for sleep problems in children (with rare exceptions, such as in the case of children with chronic conditions, such as autism, or when used for very specific circumstances, such as a long plane ride) is essentially a quick fix. We view them as a temporary way of giving children and parents some breathing room in order to get a behavioral plan in place. Sometimes parents and kids

are so stuck in the rut of bedtime struggles or so exhausted by middle-of-the night battles that they just can't see their way out. Parents in this situation often feel like they've tried everything and are not willing or are just too tired to try another behavioral strategy. Some even get to the point where they are so angry and frustrated that they have momentarily thought about hurting their child. In these cases, medication given under a doctor's supervision can reduce bedtime struggles and provide a brief respite so that parents and kids can regroup, get some catch-up sleep, and move on to really tackling the problem.

Rule 4: Sleep medication should always be combined with good sleep habits.
Don't forget the basics—including such things as having a bedtime routine, keeping a regular sleep schedule, and avoiding caffeine (see chapter 6). Stick closely to these tried-and-true sleep rules. They may not completely take care of the sleep problem, but without them you're doomed to failure.

Rule 5: Always do a trial run.
If you are considering giving your child or teenager a sleep medication for a specific short-term situation (such as a long car ride, a transatlantic flight, the night before the big dance recital), make sure you do a dry run first. Although certain side effects are common to certain medications, others are more unpredictable. In particular, Benadryl can have a paradoxical effect in some children that revs them up instead of slowing them down. The last thing you want when you arrive at Grandma's house for Thanksgiving dinner after a six-hour drive is a screaming, very cranky, and very wired child. And don't wait until the night before the exam to make sure that your teenager's sleep medication at the prescribed dose works. You could have a major meltdown on your hands.

Rule 6: "Primum non nocere."
For you non-Latin scholars out there, this basically translates as "first, do no harm." Which means if you are going to give your child a sleep medication, use one that is effective but has as few side effects as possible and that has the shortest possible duration (to avoid morning hangover or grogginess the next day). Also, use it only when needed and for the shortest possible amount of

time. Having a clear goal or endpoint in mind ("Jason will be in his own bed by 8:00 PM and fall asleep by 8:30 PM five nights out of seven") helps tremendously in making the decision as to when to stop the medication.

What about melatonin?

Melatonin has to be one of the most widely used over-the-counter sleep products. It is also one of the most misunderstood. Melatonin pills basically contain a synthetic form of a hormone that is produced in your brain in response to darkness and is turned off by light. Melatonin plays a key role in controlling a person's internal clock (see chapter 2). Therefore, it makes perfect sense to use it for circadian rhythm problems like jet lag and delayed sleep phase syndrome (see chapter 15). What does not make a whole lot of sense, however, is to use it as people generally do: for trouble falling asleep or staying asleep, which has nothing to do with a circadian problem (for how to tell the difference, see chapter 15). Melatonin has a very mild drowsiness effect (which is probably what most folks are feeling when they take it). But if you are going to take a sleep medication for insomnia, it's more logical to take one of a number of other available sleep medications that are safe and more likely to be effective.

Some people feel more comfortable using something for sleep, like melatonin, that they think of as more natural. But there are a couple of holes in this argument of which you should be aware. First, there's not a great deal of good scientific information on either the short-term or long-term safety of melatonin. For example, we know that melatonin affects the hormones that control sexual development, so this is at least a theoretical risk in using it in children. Second, the FDA does not regulate its production, so the purity and concentration of what you are getting over the counter may be suspect. Third, we have very little information about what an appropriate dose is, especially in children. Some studies have used up to ten milligrams in blind children (who often have circadian rhythm problems), while newer studies have suggested that a dose as small as one-tenth milligram (a one-hundred-fold difference!) may be effective in kids! The bottom line is, we just don't know enough yet to make solid recommendations about the use of melatonin in children and adolescents. The good news is, however, that there are a number of studies going on right now that should give us some of those answers in the next few years.

APPENDIX A

Sleep Diaries

PEDIATRIC SLEEP LOG

Child's name: _____

Child's birth date: ____ / ____ / ____

Example: Shade in the periods when you were asleep

↓ Mark your bedtime and any nap times with downward arrows. ↓

↑ Mark the time you get up in the morning and after any naps with upward arrows. ↑

Date	Day											
	1											
	2											

Date	Day	Mid night	2 AM	4 AM	6 AM	8 AM	10 AM	Noon	2 PM	4 PM	6 PM	8 PM	10 PM	Mid night

Take Charge of Your Child's Sleep

Sleep Diary

Every morning when you get up complete the sleep diary for the previous night. For example, on Monday morning fill in the information for Sunday night.

Day	Last night I went to bed at:	This morning I I woke up at:	It took me ____ minutes to fall asleep:	Total amount of sleep:
Example:				
Sunday	*12:15*	*9:20*	*25*	*9 hrs. 10min.*

APPENDIX B
Resources for Families

RESOURCES

American Academy of Sleep Medicine (AASM)
One Westbrook Corporate Center, Suite 920
Westchester, IL 60154
Phone: (708) 492-0930
Fax: (708) 492-0943
www.aasmnet.org
www.sleepeducation.com

Sleep Research Society (SRS)
One Westbrook Corporate Center, Suite 920
Westchester, IL 60154
Phone: (708) 492-0930
Fax: (708) 492-0943
www.sleepresearchsociety.org

National Sleep Foundation (NSF)
1522 K Street, NW, Suite 500
Washington, DC 20005
Phone: (202) 341-3471
Fax: (202) 341-3472
www.sleepfoundation.org

Narcolepsy Network Inc.
10921 Reed Hartman Highway
Cincinnati, OH 45242
Phone: (513) 891-3522
Fax: (513) 891-3836
E-mail: narnet@aol.com
www.narcolepsynetwork.org

Restless Legs Syndrome Foundation
819 Second St., SW
Rochester, MN 55902-2985
www.rls.org

American Sleep Apnea Association
A.W.A.K.E. Network
1424 K Street, NW, Suite 302
Washington, DC 20005
Phone: (202) 293-3650
Fax: (202) 293-3656
E-mail: asaa@sleepapnea.org
www.sleepapnea.org

National Center on Sleep Disorders Research (NCSDR)
Two Rockledge Center
Suite 7024
6701 Rockledge Drive, MSC 7920
Bethesda, MD 20892-7920
Phone: (301) 435-0199
Fax: (301) 480-3451
www.nhlbi.nih.gov/about/ncsdr/index.htm

OTHER ORGANIZATIONS

American Academy of Pediatrics
141 Northwest Point Boulevard
Elk Grove Village, IL 60007-1098
Phone: (847) 434-4000
Fax: (847) 434-8000
www.aap.org

American Psychological Association
750 First Street, NE
Washington, DC 20002-4242
Phone: (800) 374-2721 or (202) 336-5500
www.apa.org

CHADD (Children and Adults with Attention-Deficit/Hyperactivity Disorder)
8181 Professional Place
Suite 150
Landover, MD 20785
Phone: (800) 233-4050
www.chadd.org

National Institutes of Health (NIH)
Building 1
1 Center Drive
Bethesda, MD 20892
Phone: (301) 496-4000
www.NIH.gov

National Institute of Mental Health (NIMH)
Information Resources and Inquiries Branch
5600 Fishers Lane, Room 15-c-105
Rockville, MD 20807
Phone: (301) 443-4515
http://gopher.nimh.nih.gov

U.S. Consumer Product Safety Commission
Office of Information and Public Affairs
Washington, DC 20207-0001
Phone: (301) 504-0990
Fax: (301) 504-0124 or (301) 504-0025
Toll-free consumer hotline: (800) 638-2772
www.cpsc.gov

BOOKS

Parenting Books

Barkley, Russell A. *Taking Charge of ADHD: The Complete, Authoritative Guide for Parents.* 2000. New York: Guilford Press.

Barkley, Russell A., and Christine M. Benton. *Your Defiant Child: Eight Steps to Better Behavior.* 1998. New York: Guilford Press.

Brazelton, T. Berry, and Joshua D. Sparrow. *Touchpoints Three to Six: Your Child's Emotional and Behavioral Development.* 2001. Oxford: Perseus Books.

Cantor, Joanne, *"Mommy, I'm Scared": How TV and Movies Frighten Children and What We Can Do to Protect Them.* 1998. New York: Harcourt Brace.

Clark, Lynn. *SOS: Help for Parents,* 2nd. ed.. 1996. Bowling Green, KY: Parents Press.

Chansky, Tamar E. *Freeing Your Child from Anxiety: Powerful, Practical Solutions to Overcoming Your Child's Fears, Phobias, and Worries.* 2004. New York: Broadway.

Durand, V. Mark. *Sleep Better!: A Guide to Improving Sleep for Children with Special Needs.* 1998. Baltimore, MD: Brookes Publishing.

Kranowitz, Carol Stock. *The Out of Sync Child: Recognizing and Coping with Sensory Integration Dysfunction.* 1998. New York: Perigee Books.

Kurcinka, Mary Sheedy. *Raising Your Spirited Child: A Guide for Parents Whose Child Is More Intense, Sensitive, Perceptive, Persistent, and Energetic.* 1991. New York: HarperCollins.

Mindell, Jodi A. *Sleeping Through the Night* (revised): *How Infants, Toddlers, and Their Parents Can Get a Good Night's Sleep.* 2005. New York: HarperResource.

Phelan, Thomas W. *1-2-3 Magic: Effective Discipline for Children 2-12.* 1995. Glen Ellyn, IL: Child Management Inc.

Rapee, Ronald M., Susan H. Spence, Vanessa Cobham, and Ann Wignall. *Helping Your Anxious Child: A Step-By-Step Guide for Parents.* 2000. Oakland, CA: New Harbinger.

Swedo, Susan A., and Henrietta L. Leonard. *Is It "Just a Phase"? How to Tell Common Childhood Phases from More Serious Problems.* 1999. New York: Broadway Books.

Wolf, Anthony E. *"Get Out of My Life, but First Could You Drive Me & Cheryl to the Mall?": A Parent's Guide to the New Teenager, revised.* 2002. New York: Farrar, Straus, and Giroux.

Adult Sleep

Dement, William C., and Christopher Vaughn. *The Promise of Sleep: A Pioneer in Sleep Medicine Explores the Vital Connection Between Health, Happiness, and a Good Night's Sleep.* 1999. New York: Delacorte.

Hauri, Peter, and Shirley Linde. *No More Sleepless Nights.* 1996. Hoboken, NJ: Wiley.

Kryger, Meir H. *A Woman's Guide to Sleep Disorders.* 2004. New York: McGraw-Hill.

Maas, James B. *Power Sleep: The Revolutionary Program That Prepares Your Mind for Peak Performance.* 1999. New York: HarperPerennial.

Smolensky, Michael, and Lynne Lamberg. *The Body Clock Guide to Better Health: How to Use Your Body's Natural Clock to Fight Illness and Achieve Maximum Health.* 2001. New York: Owl Books.

Walsleben, Joyce A., and Rita Baron-Faust. *A Woman's Guide to Sleep: Guaranteed Solutions for a Good Night's Rest.* 2000. New York: Crown.

Wolfson, Amy R. *The Woman's Book of Sleep: A Complete Resource Guide.* 2001. Oakland, CA: New Harbinger

ACKNOWLEDGMENTS

Our gratitude first goes to all the children, adolescents, and families who have shared their stories, their dilemmas, and their sleepless nights with us.

Our appreciation also goes to those who have supported this project: agent extraordinaire Carol Mann, who was enthusiastic about the need to provide parents with information about sleep issues in older children and adolescents; and our editor, Suzanne McCloskey, for her insight about the importance of this project.

We'd also like to thank all of the many mentors and colleagues who over the years have so generously shared with us their wisdom and experience about children and sleep. We couldn't have done it without you.

And, most importantly, to our families, who have always been there for us. Our parents, who guided us and supported our drive and motivation, and who always said that there wasn't anything we couldn't do. Our husbands, for their unwavering support and patience (and for taking care of everything when we were too busy writing). And, of course, our children, who are the light of our lives and who have taught us the most about what it means to be a parent.

INDEX